To Bryan and his mother, Mary.

The day our son Bryan was born, in the first half hour while his mother was being tended to, I gave him his first Rolfing session. Every day for the next three years, he had a massage either from his mother or from me. We did everything in this book and more, and it all worked. Though we were divorced when he was two, I kept in close contact by calling at least twice a day. Mary passed away when he was ten, and I pretty much raised him on my own after that—with lots of help from friends.

The last time I worked on Bryan was at his wedding when we found ourselves together for an hour. I asked, "Do you want me to work on you a little?" and off we went. So, to this day, I can say I have never lost touch with him or he with me. In addition, he has always been willing for me to share with others what we did together to have an amazing relationship.

To my dear Bryan, for all the lessons I have learned in raising you. Here's to reaching out and bringing the power of touch to the rest of the world.

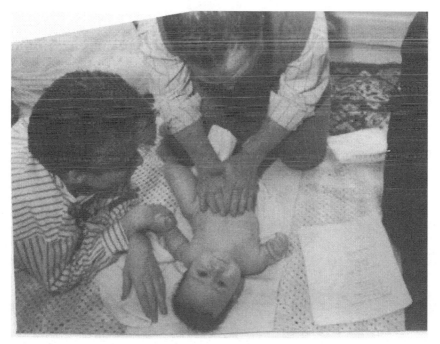

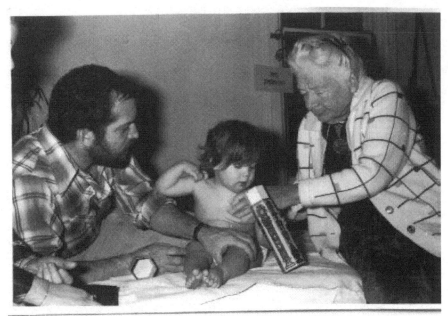

Robert Toporek, Dr. Rolf, and Shira in 1978 beginning TeamChildren.

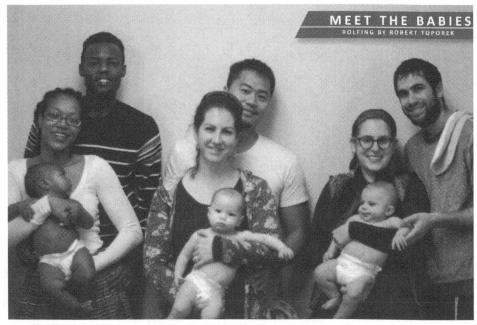

MEET THE BABIES
ROLFING BY ROBERT TOPOREK

The Nozomos, the Nguyens, and the Shinefields—new beginnings.

HANDS-ON PARENTING

A PRACTICAL GUIDE TO MASSAGE FOR HAPPIER, HEALTHIER, SMARTER KIDS

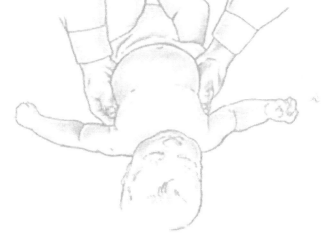

ROBERT TOPOREK

ADVANCED CERTIFIED ROLF® PRACTITIONER

Editorial work and production management: Eschler Editing
Editors: Heidi Brockbank and Michele Preisendorf
Cover design: Toby Schmidt
Interior illustrations: Lisa Adams
Book coaching: Steve Harrison and Quantum Leap
Interior print design and layout: Sydnee Hyer
eBook design and layout: Sydnee Hyer

Published by TeamChildren

First Edition: January 2018

Printed in the United States of America

10   9   8   7   6   5   4   3   2

ISBN: 978-0-9995717-0-5
This book may be ordered directly from TeamChildren.org for $15.95 plus $2.50 for postage and handling, but try your local bookstore first.
Visit us on the web at: www.handsonparenting.org

My purpose in writing *Hands-On Parenting* is to provide a guide to massage for happier, healthier, smarter kids and to expand our Hands-on Parenting workshops, seminars, videos, and any effort toward making a difference.

This book is full of knowledge, much of which is common sense but rarely common practice. My dream is for this knowledge of touch to reach every child no matter their economic or social circumstances or place of residence. It is important for every child—especially for children living in orphanages, homeless shelters, pockets of poverty, war-torn areas, and those facing developmental challenges—to benefit from the knowledge in this book and our programs.

I initially wrote this book because Buz Teacher of Running Press asked me to, and knowing I couldn't say no, I said yes. Since then I have learned so much more about the power and importance of raising happier, healthier, and smarter kids. I could not let this knowledge go untapped. Thank you, Buz.

I have no degrees in early childhood development, medicine, or massage. This book is based on my hands-on experience of working with babies, children, and their families since 1966. It all began when I started working with children in a refugee village in Vietnam. In 1975, I had the privilege of being trained as a Rolf practitioner by Dr. Ida P. Rolf, founder, and her son, Dick Demmerle. In 1978, Dr. Rolf asked me to initiate and manage a project that would document and promote the benefits of Rolfing babies and children. Since then I have worked with kids and their parents at the top of the mountain and with kids in places you would not ordinarily visit. I hope the knowledge in this book becomes an integral part of infant and early childhood development as well as a benefit to anyone at any age.

APPRECIATION

I had the extraordinary opportunity to study under Dr. Ida P. Rolf on a regular basis over the last four years of her life. Thank you, Dr. Rolf, for your knowledge, wit, wisdom, and for trusting me to carry on your work with babies, children, and families.

To all those who have contributed to my years of work either financially, through volunteering, or by trusting me with their children's lives and bodies.

To Dick Demmerle (Dr. Rolf's son) and his family, who took me into their home, family, and hearts and gave me a start by putting my hands on babies and children, starting with their children.

To Glamour magazine for mentioning me in one sentence in an article that forever changed the trajectory of my life.

To the Ford Foundation for giving me a one-year leadership development fellowship to study methods and techniques of personal growth and its relationship to public education. This allowed me out of the constraints of then common thinking and practices.

To Esalen Institute for all the training and development to lead Gestalt and encounter groups, and to Dick Price, for his friendship and support. To Deborah Meadows, for my very first massage and for the opportunity to meet Dr. Rolf.

To Werner Erhard, and the staff, leadership, and participants of Landmark Worldwide for the many years of transformation, challenges, and support of my work in all its iterations.

To Buz Teacher at Running Press for trusting, pushing, pulling, and encouraging me all the way.

To my editor, Greg Jones, for having the uncanny ability to polish this gem and Molly Jay for her ability to see it into print.

To Jean Axelrod in Philadelphia, for her extraordinary ability to edit my writing, for taking my ideas and help shape them into a work of art, for keeping me focused, and for helping me bring this to its conclusion. Also for being able to work with me during one of the worst times of my life and sharing this body of knowledge on a global level.

To Glenn Doman and his family for the pioneering work in equipping and empowering parents of both well babies and those with developmental challenges to become the best they can be and for allowing me to learn and implement their programs with my own son and in pioneering preschool and kindergarten programs.

To Oakworks, manufacturers of massage tables, and the other massage-table manufacturers, for donating a massage table to my effort to bring the power of touch to kids living in one of Philadelphia's most distressed neighborhoods, formerly called "The Badlands of North Philadelphia."

To www.brillkids.com, www.brillbaby.com, and KL Wong for his extraordinary work to make a difference in the world with early childhood education and for his beyond-the-call-of-duty support or me and Team-Children.

This book would not have been published without the major contribution of a number of key people:

Toby Schmidt, a long time friend and client, for her wonderful cover design.

Steve Harrison and his Quantum Leap Program and his encouragement of own my expert status.

Eschler Editing for their amazing ability to work with me to completion and for their amazing editor, Heidi Brockbank.

My incredible interior book designer, Sydnee Hyer.

Lisa Adams for helping me recover these great illustrations after seventeen years.

To all my supporters of our digital inclusion project, the kids of Ninth and Indiana.

And to Deborah, who lived through my producing this book.

And to my buddies from Vietnam.

And to all the restaurants who have helped fuel our mission, including Chick-fil-A, Hooters, Wegman's Giant, Acme, Olive Garden, Oaks Pizzeria Baldini's Pizza and Pasta, Affamatos Pizza and Italian Restaurant, Champs, Chaps, Maggiano's Wayback Burgers, Frito Lay, Herr's, Burger King, Wendy's, and Home Depot, to mention a few. If we missed you on this list, you know who you are!

And finally, to my generous, anonymous landlords.

"Your children are not your children.
They are sons and daughters of Life's longing for itself.
They come through you but not from you.
And though they are with you yet they belong not to you.
You may give them your love but not your thoughts,
For they have their own thoughts.
You may house their bodies but not their souls,
For thir souls dwell in the house of tomorrow, which you
cannot visit, not even in your dreams.
You may strive to be like them, but seek not
to make them like you.
For life goes not backward nor tarries with yesterday.
You are the bows from which your children as living
arrows are sent forth.
The archer sees the mark upon the path of the infinite,
and He bends you with His might that His arrows may go
swift and far.
Let your bending in the archer's hand be for gladness.
For even as He loves the arrow that flies, so He also loves
the bow that is stable."

–KAHLIL GIBRAN

CONTENTS

TENSION

In order to appreciate massage, one must understand tension. Tension is not necessarily bad because, either consciously or unconsciously, it can send warning signals that something is amiss. However, tension keeps feelings and sensations at bay. Understanding its limiting effect, and how to counteract it, is essential in massaging your babies and children. There are two fundamental tensions that we carry in our bodies: "structural tension" and "acquired tension."

Structural tension is the tensional pattern that literally shapes how we stand, walk, sit, move, express ourselves, and experience our lives. These patterns are genetic and specific to our family background. In fact, as we grow older, people may remark that we stand or walk just like our parents do. If you can recognize a structural similarity between yourself and your parent(s), you may soon be able to recognize it in your own child.

Acquired tension comes as a result of our experiences in life—both the physical and emotional challenges we inevitably face. Our bodies respond to stress and trauma by tightening, shortening, and/or contracting muscles. Over time, these instinctual muscular reactions to stressful situations turn into the tension and the inflexibility that can cause greater problems. Moreover, as we age, these responses become more firmly ingrained and more difficult to reverse.

Life presents many forms of stress to all of us, and the best thing we can do for our children is to prepare them for it. Our first trauma is birth itself. Even though there have been tremendous advances in the facility of the birth process, such as having fathers in the delivery room and providing a comfortable and cheerful maternity suite, babies still experience shock, loss, and separation from the womb. Their bodies respond to this experience by tightening and shortening, thus initiating a pattern that, unless interrupted, will govern their growth and development.

In short, massage is your child's best defense against the damages that can be caused by tension, stress, and life's traumas. It is up to you to counteract tension right from the start by providing your child with the tools to effectively and positively deal with the stressors of life. In addition, you will be giving them positive messages about their worth and well-being.

–ROBERT TOPOREK

PREFACE

The power and importance of touch in human growth development cannot be overstated. Neuroscience is now verifying that from the moment we are conceived, our brains grow at the fastest rate until age five or six. Science has shown that touch is an essential part of our cognitive, physical, and social/emotional development.

In an article on the importance of touch, author Crystal Leonard states,

> Touch is by far the most interesting and necessary of the "five senses." Any movement requires an acute awareness of one's own body which is gained through proprioception, an internal form of tactile sense. The sense of touch develops before all other senses in embryos, and is the main way in which infants learn about their environment and bond with other people. This sense never turns off or takes a break, and it continues to work long after the other senses fail in old age. Throughout life people use their sense of touch to learn, protect themselves from harm, relate to others, and experience pleasure. Interestingly, positive touch from others is necessary for an individual's healthy development. Despite the presence of all other life requirements, without this positive touch infants will fail to thrive.

Tiffany Field, head of the Touch Research Institute at the University of Miami's Miller School of Medicine, has studied the effects of touch on human health and development for over thirty years. In one study, she and her colleagues demonstrated the powerful, positive effects of touch on premature infants.

> In their first set of studies (1986), these researchers stroked and manipulated the limbs of premature infants in a neonatal intensive care unit for fifteen minutes, three times a day, for ten days. A control group of preemies did not receive the touch therapy. Results showed that the massaged preemies gained 47% more weight, were more socially responsive, and went home 6 days sooner than did the preemies in the control group. These improvements translated into a savings of $3000 per hospital stay for preemies in the massage therapy group.

Field's research has shown impressive results across the spectrum, from premature infants to children, teens, and even adults. "Even short bursts of touch—as little as fifteen minutes in the evening, in one of her studies—not only enhance growth and weight gain in children but also lead to emotional, physical, and cognitive improvements in adults."

Other researchers have recently shown that touch has the ability to boost the immune system of people who have been exposed to the common cold. A group of over four hundred participants were exposed to the cold virus. Those who received the most hugs over the course of a day were less likely to succumb to the virus, and if they did, experienced fewer symptoms with less severity.

The studies done to date show we're just beginning to understand how vital touch is to our health and well-being. And even though there is ample research on the benefits of massage for individual babies and children, we are a long way from documenting the benefits for groups of babies and children over a long period of time. Hopefully this book will lead the way to funding this type of project.

You will learn many lessons in this book. Important lessons. Profound lessons. But most importantly, you will learn that massage—along with its vast emotional and physical benefits—is fun! It is fun for the giver and fun for the receiver. When you see your baby laughing and gurgling during and after his massage, you'll understand this.

Of course, there are other reasons to begin massaging your baby or child today—no matter what their age. Massage is one of the most important developmental tools you can use as a parent. It will help your child grow—in mind and body—more rapidly and significantly than if he were to be raised without the joy of massage. It will help prevent many of the physical and emotional tensions that many people accept as "normal." And what's more, massage will keep your family in touch—literally.

Massage has been a revered art and practiced throughout history. The ancient Egyptians, Greeks, and Romans wrote that massage fostered healing and good health. In Asian countries, massage has always formed an integral part of the medical process, and references to massage in China date back to around 3000 BC. Obviously, the art of massage has been an important aspect of the human experience for a long time, proving the incredible importance of touch for human beings.

Many studies have determined that a child deprived of touch will inevitably experience isolation and loneliness, and chances are he will not thrive nearly as well as his massaged counterpart. Babies and children need touch to survive and grow. This truth was demonstrated as early as the thirteenth century, when Emperor Frederick II of Germany conducted an experiment on a number of newborns to learn what language babies would speak if they were raised without hearing any words. The babies were secluded, and the nurses assigned to feed them were forbidden to cuddle or talk to them. The experiment was a horrible failure. Not only did the babies never learn a language, they all died before they talked at all. Undoubtedly, the total lack of tactile stimulation—of human touch—proved fatal.

Fortunately, it is a natural instinct for caring parents to caress and cuddle their babies, and children make their appreciation of touch abundantly clear through vocal response and body language. As a parent reading this book, you are already aware of this fact. But you may not be aware of the scientific research that proves this. Cross-cultural studies have indicated that when infants are held, massaged, rocked, breastfed, and carried, they become adults who are less aggressive and violent and more cooperative and compassionate. As you will discover in this book, a simple, regular massage routine—as a supplement to the loving touch parents and other family members give to a child—will prove extremely valuable in a child's life.

Though there are literally hundreds and hundreds of studies on the psychology of raising babies and children, there are fewer than a dozen or so books on massage for babies and children. And most of the books that do exist concentrate on the physical aspects of massage. This book and our Hands-on Parenting program go far beyond what is now commonly known or practiced.

According to one study, one in three children and adolescents are overweight or obese, one in sixty-eight children has been identified with autism, and the statistics go on and on. If this book does anything, it will help you be more in touch with your children. And it may possibly prevent many of the complications that plague our society.

More and more parents are becoming increasingly aware of how important massage can be for all members of the family. More and more magazines and newspapers have begun to extol the virtues of massage for babies.

National television and radio programs have also gotten into the act, featuring segments in which babies are massaged while doctors enthusiastically list all the wonderful benefits a regularly massaged child will reap in his life.

Many regard such segments with surprise and sometimes humor, because they consider regular massage to be something only the wealthy indulge in—via the services of an expensive, professional masseur or masseuse—as a luxury. But those who try it themselves quickly learn that massaging your baby and/or child is not just a novelty . . . it's a necessity. For the thousands of parents who have established a regular massage program for their children, massage has become an essential component of good parenting. They have learned that the top ingredients are a healing touch and an open heart.

Indeed, massage offers tremendous benefits. It can become one of the most important tools you'll ever use as a parent, enhancing your relationship with your children while providing more pleasure from that interaction than you can imagine. Starting a massage program early in a child's life is an important step in forestalling future problems, both physical and emotional.

Fear of touch, poor body image, lack of body awareness, and high levels of tension are just some of the negative effects that stem from a lack of nurturing touch during childhood. Massage during the formative years is a powerful way to teach your child positive lessons about touch, intimacy, and body awareness. Physically, massage stretches the soft tissues, relieves muscle spasms, facilitates movement of bodily fluids (blood and lymph), and stimulates the nervous system. Massage also encourages the production of a number of vital hormones, including the growth hormone somatotropin. Emotionally, massage fosters positive feelings about body awareness and about interpersonal touch.

Despite extensive research and the commonsense knowledge of the benefits of massage for physical and mental development in babies and children, it has not become common practice. Far too often, not enough is being done to take full advantage of this brief but essential window of time.

Over the decades I have worked with babies and children using the massage techniques in this book, the ancillary tips at the end of every chapter, and Rolfing babies, children, and families since 1975, I've seen hundreds of success stories, including a young woman with Down syndrome who, due to the diligence of her parents in exploring all possible ways to provide opportunities for her full development, was able to graduate with a college degree in dance and theatre.

This book is about more than just massaging babies and children. It's about the ancillary things you can do to support cognitive and neurological development. Massage is a powerful tool, but when parents incorporate the additional exercises included in each section, it is greatly magnified, and the result can be quantum leaps and bounds in a child's development and success in life.

Our intention is that this book will raise awareness of the power of massage and help children all over the world reach their fullest potential.

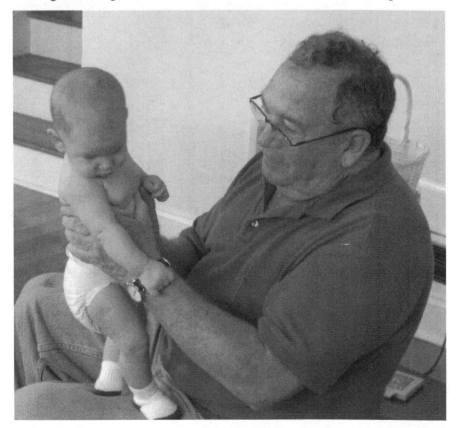

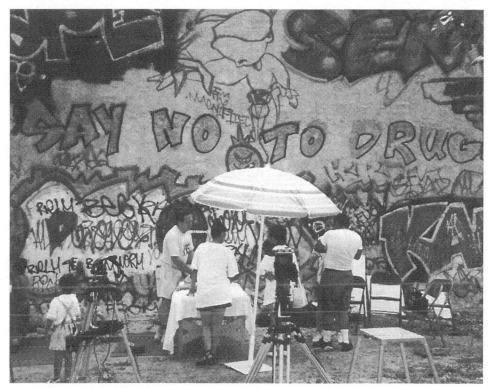

Taking massage/Rolfing to the streets of North Philadelphia.

"If a child is to keep alive his inborn sense of wonder without any such gift from the fairies, he needs the companionship of at least one adult who can share it, rediscovering with him the joy, excitement and mystery of the world we live in."

–RACHEL CARSON

INTRODUCTION

Parents worldwide have always used minor massage techniques to treat their children's common aches and pains. One may rub an area that has received an impact to keep a bruise from swelling. Mother may rub her baby's tender gums during teething to relieve discomfort. Dad may massage away his child's nighttime leg-muscle cramps—known as "growing pains"—to soothe her and help her sleep. It is no surprise that the soothing touch of a parent has always been extremely important to the healthy development of children.

However, such wonderful touch has traditionally been employed only as a reactive treatment for an ache or pain. The time has come to realize that touch—in particular, a regular massage strategy—can be used as a preventive measure against the negative stresses and tensions of life.

Formal massage for babies was only recently recognized in America with the founding of the University of Miami's Touch Research Institute in 1992. Studies show that premature babies who were massaged daily fared significantly better than preemies that were not massaged. Full-term babies, when massaged even for short periods, have been found to sleep better and have less colic difficulties and other ailments common to newborns than their unmassaged counterparts. Long-term effects have proven more significant in terms of positive mental and physical development.

After all, this book is primarily about possibilities. Sit down and think about what you want for your baby, yourself, and your family. You want good mental, physical, and spiritual health for your loved ones and yourself. Massage offers infinite possibilities to help you achieve those goals. Massage, with its mixture of love, compassion, and common sense, will play a vital role in maintaining that precious good health.

Classes teaching massage for babies are springing up around the country. Although these classes are instructive, you do not need formal training to give your child the gift of a loving massage. You will, however, benefit from learning the accepted techniques of massage that are employed by professional massage therapists. This book will take you, step-by-step, to each part of the body—from between each toe to the top of the head. You will find that massage can actually be quite simple, and eventually—with these basic techniques as a foundation—you will learn to improvise your own techniques! Your child will express her pleasure or displeasure with the way she is touched, just as your hands will become accustomed to the unique shape of her body and the sensations that give her the most benefits. The exercises in this book are geared toward different age groups, or children at different stages of life. Every child is different, so use your judgment as to which activities will be most beneficial for your child.

Massage is often thought of as a luxury, or as something that is used after a problem arises. Yet you'll soon see that massage can be done by anyone, to anyone else, at any time. This book is written for every family member. Grandmothers love to massage babies while mothers tend to other chores. Older children can massage the younger. The young child herself, with her soft little hands, can derive pleasure from massaging those who first massaged her. And to all the dads out there, you'll see that this book is aimed at you every bit as much as to your baby's mother. The purpose of this book is to encourage, empower, and equip every family member to use massage as a powerful tool in counteracting the stresses and strains of life.

This book has been arranged in an easy-to-use format. Part One offers some preliminary tips on getting started. You will become familiar with the various tools necessary for a successful massage, including where to massage, which oils to use, and other tips and hints. Part One also addresses the problem of tension—what it means to us as human beings, how it develops, and what effects it may have on our bodies and minds.

In part two, you will learn professional massage techniques as they apply to specific body areas. This part is separated into ten sections: chest and shoulders, legs and feet, sides of the body, inner legs, abdomen, extensor muscles, head and neck, lower body, upper body, and connecting the body. Although at first these groupings may seem arbitrary and repetitive, you will soon see that this important arrangement will make it easier for you to tackle small areas at a time. Also, this structure will give you a unique chance to discover and appreciate how the parts of the body are interconnected, and how they function as a whole. Tips are provided throughout to assist you in talking to your child regarding the significance of each part of the body. Then she, too, will understand how she can utilize each part most efficiently.

Also included with each body area is a corresponding philosophy on an important life aspect, essential for maximum integration of mind and body. This will help your child develop a healthy awareness of the connection between her inner and outer being.

Part three addresses special concerns and the important groundbreaking work of TeamChildren.org in taking these ideas and out into the world we live in.

As you'll soon find out, this book is unusual in a number of different ways. Whereas most books have a beginning, middle, and end, the "ending" in this book is instead a continuation. Massage for children is an ongoing experience and every day is a new beginning. Also, whereas most books on massage concentrate on technique and the physiological impacts of massage, this book treats mind and body as one.

So let this book teach you the simple techniques that can transform how you relate to and raise your child. In the process, you'll learn a good deal more about yourself as well. You'll also become so aware of the inestimable value of massage that you'll probably seek out a massage therapist for yourself! Or even better, you'll soon be recruiting family members to massage you and each other. You'll be a family that's truly "in touch" in every way!

There are countless examples of specific, measurable benefits to the child, who is massaged on a regular basis, including:

- Improved motor development
- Faster bodily growth
- Improved breathing
- Improved circulation
- Less agitation
- Less pain from gas and constipation
- Greater poise and response in social situations
- Release of accumulated tension
- Overall, a happier child

DISCOVER HOW MANY MORE BENEFITS YOU CAN ADD TO THIS LIST!

We in the Western world are beginning to discover our neglected senses. This growing awareness represents something of an overdue insurgency against the painful deprivation of sensory experience we have suffered in our technologized world. The ability of Western man to relate to his fellowman has lagged far behind his ability to relate to consumer goods and the unnecessary necessities which hold him in thrall possessed by his possessions. He can reach out to other planets, but too often he cannot reach out to his fellowman. His personal frontiers seldom, if at all, permit the passage of a deeply felt communication across them. The human dimension is constricted and constrained. Through what other media, indeed, than our senses can we enter into that healthy tissue of human contacts, the universe of human existence. We seem to be unaware that it is our senses that frame the body of our reality.

To shut off any one of the senses is to reduce the dimensions of our reality, and to the extent that that occurs we lose touch with it; we become imprisoned in a world of impersonal words, sans touch, sans taste, sans flavor. The one dimensionality of the word becomes a substitute for the richness of the multidimensionality of the senses, and our world grows crass, flat, and arid in consequence. Words tend to take the place of experience. Words become a declarative statement rather than a demonstrative involvement, something one can utter in words, rather than act out in a personal sensory relationship.

Above all else, it seems to me that is our role as human beings always to join learning to loving kindness. Learning to learn, learning to love, and to be kind are so closely interconnected and so profoundly interwoven, especially with the sense of touch, it would greatly help toward our rehumanization if we would pay closer attention to the need we all have for tactual experience.

The impersonality of life in the Western world has become such that we have produced a race of untouchables. We have become strangers to each other, not only avoiding but even warding off all forms of "unnecessary" physical contact, faceless figures in a crowded landscape, lonely and afraid of intimacy. To the extent that this is so, we are all diminished. Because of our untouchableness we have failed to create a society in which people touch each other in more senses than the physical. With our inauthentic selves, and wearing other people's image of what we should be, it is not surprising that we remain unsure of who we really are. We wear the inauthentic selves that have been imposed upon us as uncomfortably as an ill fitting garment, ruefully, at times, and unknowing, wondering how we got this way. As Willy Loman says in Death of a Salesman, "I still feel kind of temporary."

PREFACE 3RD EDITION *TOUCHING* by ASHLEY MONTAGU

PART ONE
GETTING STARTED

NEVER UNDERESTIMATE THE INTELLIGENCE OF YOUR BABY! Babies and young children are infinitely smarter than adults usually acknowledge, and they have an incredible capacity to learn new things. Scientific research continues to reveal the important benefits of physical and verbal stimulation for infants. Some doctors and research specialists even assert that this stimulation begins in the womb. It is up to you to provide your child with all the positive and useful information you can.

When you begin to massage your child, you should realize that each touch, each stroke, each tickle, and each word you offer him will be accepted, understood, and put on file in his little mind. The more you speak to him, the more he will understand the world around him. More importantly, your child will become infinitely smarter the more you massage him. That's because you'll be banishing the tension that can literally block his mental and physical development, and you'll be stimulating all the bodily functions to work in concert. The mind-body connection will become increasingly apparent as you become more adept at massage.

There are many different schools of massage—many requiring years of study of anatomy and physiology. Most of these schools have developed to meet the needs of people whose bodies have stored up years of tension.

Yet the field of massaging newborns, toddlers, and young children has not grown apace, perhaps because stress in someone so young cannot be fully appreciated. However, tension does exist in babies and children. Birth itself is the first real trauma we must survive and our first break from the safe and comfortable environment of our mother's womb, where all our needs were met. More importantly, there is certainly the potential to develop stress in this life. Trials and tribulations abound all around us—from broken or dysfunctional families, to school bullying, to financial hardship, to health problems, to the violence in Chicago, to the war-torn nations of the world, to the challenges of poverty faced around the globe. Nurturing your child through massage can provide relief from these tensions and give them a better life. Perhaps the greatest benefit of massaging babies and children is to lay a foundation of growth and development that will prevent these tensions from taking a stronghold in your child's life.

Many people have a preconceived notion of what a massage is. They picture a thirty-minute session involving rubbing and poking and stretching and kneading. The person giving the massage is usually very structured and professional. The person being massaged is usually quiet and still—as if they are not actively participating in the process. Well, throw out all of those notions, because massaging your baby and child does not have to fit any stereotype of "what a massage should be." On the following pages are four quick tips to help you develop an attitude about massage that works for you and your family.

The Bumblebee Cannot Fly ... According to recognized aerotechnical tests, the bumblebee cannot fly because of the shape and weight of his body in relation to the total wing area.

But, the bumblebee doesn't know this so he goes ahead and flies anyway.

TIPS

1. K.I.S.S. (KEEP IT SHORT AND SIMPLE, MAKE IT FUN)

You don't need to be professionally trained in massage techniques to provide your child with a wonderful massage experience. You need not massage the entire body each time you massage your child. And your technique does not have to be sophisticated or refined. The major requirements are that you be a loving parent, that you have common sense, and that you keep it simple. It doesn't take very long to make a huge difference to your child. Remember that this is your baby, and he will be getting to know your touch. At the same time, you'll be learning what feels good to him as you learn more about his body.

The most important aspect of massage for a newborn is the experience of contact. So keep it short until he grows a bit. A five or ten-minute massage stimulates a newborn to the extent that an hour-long massage does an adult. This instructional section of this book (Part 2) provides massage techniques for different areas of the body. You may choose to massage the arms and shoulder one day and the legs and feet another time. This is perfectly acceptable!

Keep it simple and use common sense. Think of what feels good to you and see if it feels good to your baby. You'll know by the way he smiles and gurgles.

2. HAVE FUN

Make massaging your baby/child is one of the most delightful things you will ever do in your life. You know your baby will not be a baby forever (thank God!), so enjoy every single moment. They are moments to be cherished.

Throughout the book, you will find plenty of tips to make the massage experience a very personal and enjoyable one. You can play games with your baby's toes and fingers, sing little songs, and tell quick stories. Most importantly, you want your baby to have fun. Be excited when you massage him. Talk to him during the massage; encourage him to giggle. Let your enthusiasm be contagious.

3. ALLOW THE INTIMACY

Massage is a very emotional experience! What I have discovered in my many years of body and transformational work is that humans are, by nature, self-protective. I know this because throughout my own life I have had to work on being more open. On a physical level, our flexor muscles, which contract and overpower the muscles that allow us to open and extend, are a built-in, inherited pattern from the moment of conception. It's simply part of being human to have a tendency to hold on, clam up, and protect ourselves based on the last time we got hurt either physically or emotionally.

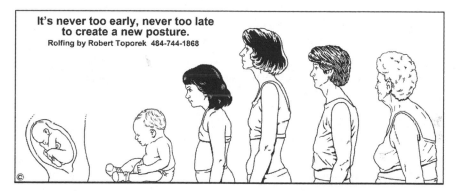

It's never too early, never too late to create a new posture.
Rolfing by Robert Toporek 484-744-1868

So before you begin massaging your child, it's a good idea to analyze yourself and identify any tensions you may be holding in. Let go of those tensions in whatever way works for you—stretching exercises, a brisk walk, listening to music, meditation. You need to relieve your own tension before you can help your child deal with his.

The opportunity to improve life through baby and child massage is invaluable for both parent and child. You will be passing to your child new messages of love, nurturing, self-confidence, communication—things you may not have inherited from your own parents. To gain a rapport with your baby, dysfunctional patterns must be changed, and you are the one who can create a new model for relating through the power of touch. You can devote much of your energy in getting to know his body and his personality. And in the process, he'll get to know you—your touch, your scent, your energy. This early intimacy can bless you and your child throughout life and affect change through generations.

So allow the intimacy—allow your thoughts, feelings, hesitations, and confidence to be expressed. Most importantly, allow your love to express itself. It will be profoundly appreciated.

4. TALK TO YOUR BABY NO MATTER HOW SILLY IT SEEMS

Babies are smarter than you think. Though she may not understand language, your baby understands what you are saying. By opening up the lines of communication through language and touch, you enable a freedom to communicate that will help both you and your child experience life to the fullest. This is an important tool your child can use with everyone he meets as he advances through school and a career and, one day, his own parenthood. Moreover, you will become a clearinghouse—as well as a safe house—for his trials and tribulations. Raise a child who is in touch with his body and emotions, and you make it possible for your child to experience life with less emotional baggage simply by bolstering his ability to express himself right from the start.

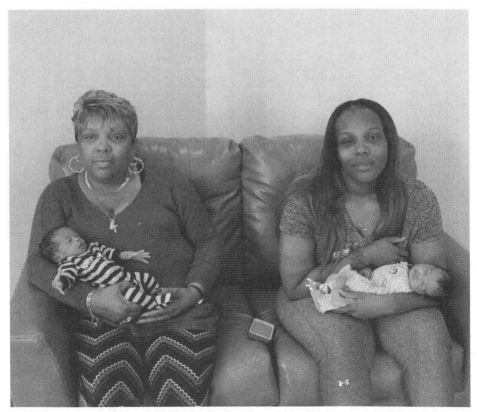

Elaine Johnson, her daughter, and new twin grandsons.

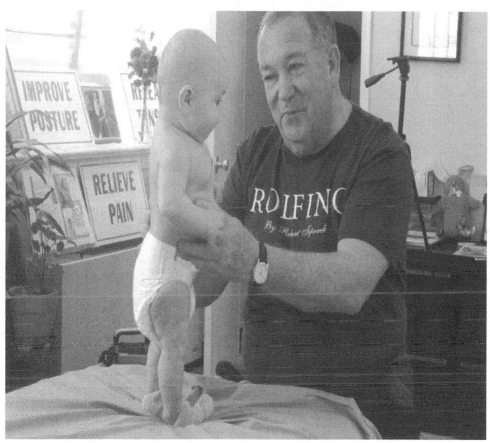

Three-month-old Colton Burke after 10 sessions.

"Education is the great engine of personal development. It is through education that the daughter
of a peasant can become a doctor, that a son of a
mineworker can become the head of the mine,
that a child of farm workers can become the
president of a nation."

–NELSON MANDELA

TOOLS
EVERYTHING YOU NEED
FOR A GREAT MASSAGE

1. SELF-AWARENESS

It is important for you to be completely familiar with your own body. Think about how your hands, fingers, feet, and toes are central to the functioning of your body. Your ankles, knees, hips, wrists, elbows and shoulders are essential for flexibility. Your head and torso are central to your relaxation and are, in fact, the locus of your entire being. Without intimate knowledge of the body's structure and function you cannot explore your baby with any success. Learn how your body feels. How does it move? What's too tight or too loose? What anxieties and tensions can you let go of? Self-awareness will become one of your most powerful tools. And remember that babies are highly intuitive; they know if all is not right with your body and your being.

2. YOUR HANDS

Your baby's skin is very sensitive so remove your rings and make sure your fingernails are cut short. Needless to say, your hands should be immaculately clean.

Each time, before beginning your massage, explore and stimulate your own hands, fingers, and fingertips. They are the primary tools you'll be using on your baby. Gently rub your fingertips together. See how softly you can make contact and then increase the pressure until it gets too hard. Feel the contours. Explore the crevices. Use your fingers in different ways, seeing how many variations in pressure you can create. Remember that no one is judging you.

Then use the fingertips of one hand to experiment with massaging the other hand. Explore all the nooks and crannies of that hand, especially the joints. When you massage, you can use the palm of your hand, the back of your hand, or the side extending from your little finger down to your wrist bone. Or, you can use the area between the thumb and fingers for some strokes. Your wrists and forearms will be used in different ways to produce different sensations. But ultimately, your fingertips will be doing most of the work.

3. MASSAGE OIL

An important element of massage is the selection and use of oils. The purpose of using oil is to reduce friction, thus allowing your hands to glide gently over your child's body without pulling or stretching the skin. Babies and toddlers alike enjoy the smooth sensation of oil. However, although oil is recommended, you do not absolutely have to use it. You may instead want to use a light dusting of talcum powder, or nothing at all.

Many therapists recommend using only cold-pressed vegetable oils such as almond, sesame, sunflower, or safflower. These oils are gentle and contain vitamins and minerals that will help nurture and moisturize your baby's skin. Any one of these oils can be readily found in most health food stores. Since babies are highly sensitive to smell, it is suggested that you use unscented oil for your first massages. When she becomes a toddler, however, your child may enjoy the sweet aromas of almond, coconut, apricot kernel, or a variety of other oils.

If you do not want to use a fruit or vegetable oil, you can use a commercial "baby oil," such as Johnson & Johnson™ Baby Oil or Baby Lotion.

Whichever kind of oil you choose, make sure to watch your baby's skin for any adverse reaction. Some babies may exhibit a slight allergic reaction to nut oils. If this happens, simply switch to safflower or avocado oil.

You may want to keep your oil in a plastic squeeze bottle. As you will use the bottle frequently during a massage, this will help prevent spills and accidents. (Others prefer to pour their oil into a bowl or other container before beginning the massage.) It is important to be sure that the oil is warmed before applying it to any part of your baby's body. You can do this one of several ways.

The easiest way is to rub the oil briskly in your hands, warming it with friction. It is also convenient to warm oil by setting the bottle in a bowl of hot water. Or you can pop it into the microwave for a few seconds—just be sure to test the temperature first! You do not want the oil to be too hot. Also remember never to pour the oil directly onto the skin—always rub it into your hands and fingertips first, and then apply it to your baby from your hands.

There are two main types of oils: base oils and essential oils. Base oils are the most common and the mildest. These base oils, namely cold-pressed vegetable and/or fruit oils, will be the ones you'll probably prefer to use on your baby's precious skin. Some examples of good base oils to use are:

- Vegetable oil
- Sunflower oil
- Safflower oil
- Grape-seed oil
- Almond oil
- Soya oil
- Peach oil
- Apricot kernel oil
- Coconut oil
- Sesame oil
- Canola oil

And if the oil you chose is enhanced with vitamin E, it's even better!

Essential oils are more concentrated. These oils must be blended with a base oil to avoid stinging sensitive skin. It is not recommended that any essential oil be used when massaging a newborn baby. As your child grows older, however, you may want to experiment with the different scents that essential oils offer.

It has been proven that various scents can have a powerful effect on both our physical health and our emotional moods. The scent of spiced apples, for example, has been shown to lower blood pressure. Other smells, such as plum or peach, can reduce pain. Jasmine and peppermint can lift depression. Geranium and bergamot help to dispel anxiety. And rose and carnation have been shown to restore energy.

You can employ scented essential oils to enhance the type of massage you want to give your child (invigorating, relaxing, etc.). Be sure to add only a few drops of the essential oil to the base oil, and mix well. Between five and ten drops should do the trick. Some essential oils you may consider are:

CHAMOMILE—this oil has a fruity, apple-like scent and is good for calming and soothing the nerves. It is also suitable for sensitive skins.

LAVENDER—this fresh-scented oil is known for its calming properties. It is also beneficial in treating headaches, insomnia, depression, aches, pains, wounds, and insect bites. Use this scent and your little one will drift off into a sweet slumber in no time.

NEROLI (ORANGE BLOSSOM)—this oil has a sweet, orange scent. It is a calming oil that helps reduce anxiety and counteract insomnia; and it is especially suited for dry skin.

MARJORAM—this "green"-scented oil is warming and comforting. It has been used to treat aches and pains, insomnia, and headaches. It is also excellent after exercise, as it increases local blood circulation.

EUCALYPTUS—a fresh, tangy, and stimulating scent that can be used for treating coughs and colds.

ROSEMARY—with a sharp herb scent, this oil is known to help stimulate memory and clear thinking. It's also useful in treating rheumatic pain, as well as aches and pains after exercise.

4. MASSAGE AREA

A steady surface is recommended. If you don't have a professional massage table, don't worry. You will find that a kitchen table, dining room table, or even a firm bed will suffice. If you're using your kitchen or dining room table, be sure that it is well padded with blankets and towels to provide a comfortable, soft surface. Also, it's a good idea to have extra towels handy in case your over-relaxed child naturally relieves himself, and also to sop up extra oil. Always be sure to use clean, fresh towels under your baby.

5. ROOM TEMPERATURE

A naked baby will feel the cold far sooner than you will, so be sure your room temperature is at least seventy degrees and that there are no drafts. A hot bath may also be an excellent way for the baby to warm up and relax, and while in the tub you can start the massage using a mild soap instead of oil.

6. QUIET TIME

Soft lighting and freedom from interruption are not vital to a successful massage, although they can make for a wonderful experience. Remember, you'll be talking to your child throughout the massage, and the line of communication will be best served in a quiet atmosphere. Bedtime is an ideal for initiating massage because the sleep area will already be warm and quiet. Of course massage also promotes restful sleep. What better time to calm a restless child!

7. YOUR BABY'S/CHILD'S ATTITUDE

A baby or toddler in pain has other priorities than a massage. Wait until you are sure the child is emotionally ready for his massage. Because you've opened up a strong line of communication, you'll recognize the signals he sends when he is ready for your loving touch.

It is always best to tell your baby ahead of time when you are going to give him a massage. About an hour before, tell your child, "Okay, a little while after lunch (dinner, playtime, etc.) we are going to have a great massage." It is a wise idea to plan the massage for a time when it is relatively calm in your house and after your baby has had time to relax from his last activity. This way you are not trying to give a massage to a distracted baby. And you will find that he will be more interested and cooperative when you give the massage.

8. YOUR ATTITUDE

Right from the start, he's an intuitive little guy who can read your moods and feel your tensions. Make sure you are in a happy mood, let your tensions go, and make sure your hands are soft and pliant. Most of all make sure you are as comfortable as he is, physically and emotionally. Your body plays an important part of your massage. One of the best things to do before you begin to massage your baby or child is to pay attention to your own tension.

Because breathing is essential to relaxing, the first thing you want to do is to pay attention to your own breathing. Pay attention to how deep it is, how fast or slow, and how much effort you are putting into it. Once you have become conscious of your own breathing, you will be in a better position to recognize your baby's breathing. It's best to evaluate your breathing patterns while lying on your back (although it can also be done sitting in a chair or even standing up). Pay attention to the rise and fall of your lungs while breathing normally. Notice any negative thoughts you may have as the breath flows into and out of your lungs. Begin to let go of these attitudes, tensions, and negative thoughts. Let a new flow of fresh air breathe new life into your whole body. The process takes just a few minutes, but is well worth the effort. Your baby will reap the benefits!

9. YOUR PROGRAM

Today it seems that parents have more to do and less time to do it. The best thing about massaging your baby and/or child is that it doesn't take very long to complete a successful massage. Babies should be massaged for five to ten minutes and toddlers can be given ten to twenty minute massages. The most important thing, though, is to create a regular massage program that both you and your child can count on. The frequency of your massages can occur anywhere from twice a day to once a week—whatever works for you and your family.

It is helpful to set some sort of schedule or program for massage. Having a routine will make things easier for both you and your baby. You will be sure to have the time, and your baby will know what to expect. You may, for example, want to begin and/or end his day with a massage. Morning is a particularly great time for massage. A morning massage will help stimulate circulation, get oxygen to the brain, increase alertness, and prepare your child for a great day. At night, you can help ease your child into sweet dreams with a soothing, relaxing massage.

The type of massage you want to give (whether invigorating or relaxing) determines the type of stroke you should use.

When your child is a bit older, a great time for massage is after school.

This is an excellent way for your child to relax and let go of stress she may have accumulated in the course of her day. It also a good time for you to talk and connect with each other. What did she learn in school today? What are his favorite subjects? What are her plans for the evening? And be sure to tell him about your day. What did you do at work/home while he was in school? What do you have planned for this evening?

If your child is on a sports team, another great time for massage is after practice. Massage will alleviate muscle aches and pains, and it will help improve performance with increased body awareness and flexibility.

Whatever schedule you come up with will be determined by the daily responsibilities of your family. Be sure to schedule your massage session at a time when it will not be interrupted or rushed. And also, be sure to stick to it!

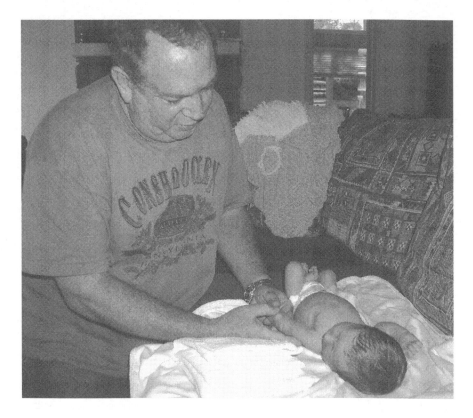

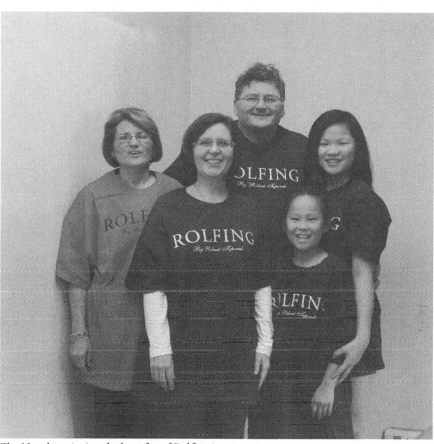

The Novaks enjoying the benefits of Rolfing/massage.

"In their freedom, birds make expanding
circles in the sky.

How do they learn to be free?

They fall—and by falling are given wings to fly."

—RUMI

PART TWO
MASSAGE INSTRUCTION

A S THE OLD SONG GOES, "The knee bone is connected to the thigh bone, the thigh bone is connected to the hip bone," and so forth. In order to help you learn how to massage your baby or child most effectively, this part of the book is divided into specific body areas. So don't feel responsible to read this entire book at once, or that you have to give a full-body massage at every session.

You—and your child—will be better served if you first become familiar with the various areas of the body individually.

Each body area in this part of the book is defined as a physical area (chest and shoulders, legs and feet, etc.). However, each of these areas is further explained in terms of its spiritual and/or emotional importance (the essence of life, our stance in life, etc.). By synthesizing this information, you will come to understand the importance of each body area in its own right and as an important part of the whole.

At first, you should massage each body area separately. This will come in handy when just the feet, legs, arms, back, or other specific area needs special attention.

Children will experience growing pains. It's part of getting older. Through play, participation in sports, and through accidents, they will also experience deep bruising to their arms, ribs, elbows, and knees. And I'm sure you know from experience how tension can create discomfort in the neck and shoulders and throughout your body.

What a gift it is to be able to focus on all these particular areas in order to massage the pains away before they lead to greater problems!

To get started, read a section on an individual body area and then work with that area of your child's body a couple of times—or until you become comfortable with the process. Then move on to the next area. Each part of the body presents an opportunity for you to develop solid massage techniques that are specific to that area. Your devoted experimentation and practice will reap big rewards—experimentation will lead you in the right direction, while practice will enhance your confidence and competence (issues that are as important to your child's well-being as they are to your own).

Once you've become familiar with each of the body areas, and are confident with your ability in each area, you will want to try a full body massage. This is covered in the last body area section of part two. By then, you will have gained an important understanding of the body as a whole.

Finally, each body area is further broken down into two sections—infants and young children. Each of these sections helps direct your efforts to your child at a particular stage of development, and also provides examples of the kind of results you can expect at each stage:

Chest and Shoulders—The Essence of Life

Legs and Feet—Our Stance in Life

Sides of the Body   The Many Sides of Life

The Inner Legs—Vitality

Abdomen   Power and Confidence

The Extensor Muscles—Extending Yourself

Head and Neck—A New Perspective

Lower Body Balance and Being in the Present

Upper Body Self-Esteem

Connecting the Body Completion

CHEST AND SHOULDERS
THE ESSENCE OF LIFE

Breathing is fundamental. It brings essential oxygen into our lungs and blood. Yet we don't usually think about the implications of our breathing since it is an automatic bodily function that we take for granted. However, it is important to understand that breathing does more than simply keep us alive; it also influences how we live. By consciously controlling one's breathing, a person may prevent tension from taking hold of the body.

We often say such things as, "We need to breathe new life into this project" or, "We need a breath of fresh air." When we want someone to slow down, we may say, "Take a breather." These common expressions reflect our unconscious knowledge that breathing is important for more than the obvious reason. Just think how much more clearly you think and feel after you "take a breather . . ."

Life is full of challenges, and challenges usually come with a good helping of tension. It is clear that unguarded tension negatively affects breathing. Fortunately, it is also clear that consciously controlled breathing reduces the effect of tension on the body, mind, and spirit.

Possibly the most important areas on your child's body to massage are the site of her breathing (lungs) and the center of her life force (heart). When you massage your child's chest area, you will promote normal breathing and give a jump-start to her circulatory system. By increasing the function of these bodily systems, you'll also be increasing brain function. Studies of newborns who were lucky enough to be massaged have shown a stronger connection between mental acuity and bodily function. Don't forget, you are your child's guide to understanding her body and the new world around her—it's a big but joyous responsibility!

For every baby, the traumatic experience of birth—leaving the comfort and security of the womb to emerge into the great big world—is unquestionably the beginning of stress. You as a parent can comfort her and ease her fears right away with your gentle touch, soothing voice, and welcoming manner. The child who is not stroked and touched early on will begin the process of holding in emotions. This emotional pitfall is manifested by a subtle contracting of muscles—a tightening of her body that will ultimately affect her breathing and her ability to relax. Eventually, if allowed to go unchecked, this contracting of muscles can cause her to erect barriers against people and life situations, and may be the first ill-advised step toward poor posture.

You may be able to see these patterns in your own life. When you are tense and stressed, you are inclined to keep even the closest family and friends at arm's length. What's more, you may react negatively to even the most pleasurable situations. When you counteract stress and tension, however—through studied breathing, massage, or other means—the improvement in all your relationships is astounding.

There are two basic ways of dealing with life's stresses: reacting and responding. Reacting is the instinctive way to deal with stress; it is an unconscious action. In massage, "reacting" means tightening up when confronted with something unpleasant. It is almost impossible to prevent oneself from reacting to stress since reaction is, by definition, your initial unconscious response to something. However, although reacting is an important function of stress control, it is unhealthy to rely on reacting as your only form of stress control. To do so would lead to the development of an uptight, inward-looking personality.

Responding is a more positive, more controlled way to handle stress. It is a conscious approach to stressful situations, and it should always follow reacting. You begin to respond when you gain control of your breathing—then, you come to an understanding of the situation and prepare yourself to face it. Responding requires a letting go, a flowing with the situation. It's a way of consciously guiding yourself to the result you want. It requires being in touch with your body and letting it be an integral part of your interactions with people and situations, whether they are adverse or pleasant. What better time is there to start teaching your child this lesson than in the beginning?

Consider the relationship between self-expression and posture. When people are fully self-expressed, they usually stand up straighter and breathe easier. They hold their shoulders back and have nothing to hide. However, human beings are defensive by nature, and many people grew up being taught to keep quiet and to speak only when spoken to. This barrier against self-expression inevitably leads to bad posture and a host of other physical and emotional problems. Our ability or inability to express ourselves affects the way we feel, the decisions we make, the jobs we choose, and every single aspect of our lives.

Think how healthy your child will become if she learns to be self-confident, self-aware, and self-assertive at an early age…You can help her achieve this level of health by teaching her to dissolve her tensions and keep them at bay—and a big part of this lesson can be taught through regular massage. She will learn to express herself more fully throughout life.

Naturally, every child has her share of falling down and getting hurt—both literally and figuratively. One of the best ways to help your child deal with any kind of trauma is first to get her to breathe and relax. It doesn't happen immediately, but after holding her for a few minutes and talking softly and reassuringly, she'll get over her upset and experience comfort at the same time. When she is able to break the bonds of tension, she'll have learned to deal with upsets in a mature, positive way.

When you massage your baby or child's chest and shoulders, you will be instilling in her very positive thoughts about breathing, posture, expression, and confidence.

HOW TO MASSAGE YOUR BABY'S/CHILD'S CHEST AND SHOULDERS

APPROXIMATE MASSAGE TIME: 3–5 MINUTES

First, put some oil on your hands and rub them together briskly until they and the oil are warmed. This warmth feels good to your baby, helping to relax her entire neuromuscular system, and no doubt it reminds her of the warmth and comfort of the womb. Nothing inhibits relaxation more than cold hands and cold oil. Spread the oil gently and evenly across her chest and shoulders.

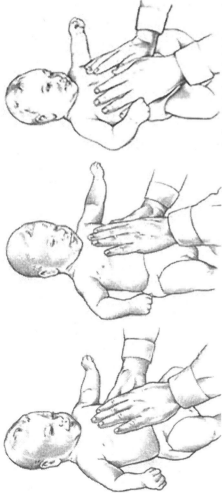

1 Lay her on her back, with her feet toward you as you stand in front of her. Place both your hands gently on her chest with your palms down and thumbs together. Then move your hands to each side, slowly and with a feather-light touch, until your fingers gently wrap around each side of her rib cage. Let your hands linger there and feel the rhythm of her breathing.

2 Place your right hand on her left side just under the rib cage. During this part of the massage, your left hand should rest very lightly on the right side of her torso, just above the waist, to give her an added sense of stability. Glide your right palm up toward her shoulders, but pause for a couple seconds to feel the beating of her heart.

3 Still using your right hand, move your palm in a light, circular motion over the area of her left lung. Hold your hand there for another few seconds to get a feel for her breathing. (And if there's a bit of congestion in her lungs, a gentle massage can help loosen the phlegm.)

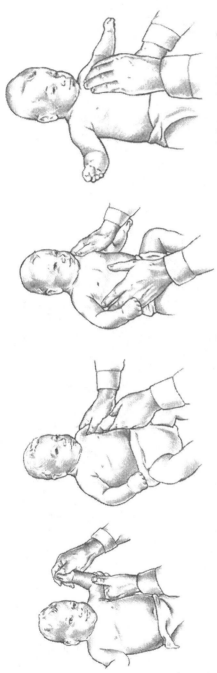

4 With the four fingertips of your right hand together, inch your way up to her collarbone. Trace the collarbone out to her left shoulder and flick your fingertips off her shoulder to release any tension.

5 Add some more oil to your hands if necessary and rub them together. Wrap your fingers around her shoulder and, applying very light pressure, grip the shoulder with your entire hand. Hold the shoulder inside your palm for several moments, gently squeezing and releasing it. (As she grows aware of her shoulder through subsequent massages, she will know how to respond when you tell her to straighten her shoulders and be aware of her posture.)

6 Wrap your hand around her arm and slowly slide it down, squeezing gently as you go until you reach her elbow. Linger there a few seconds so she can become aware of her elbow joint, then continue on in the same fashion until you reach the wrist. Again linger there, rubbing your fingers back and forth over her wrist and the top of her hand. Make tiny circular motions on the back of her hand until you reach her fingers. Finish by pulling each finger and the thumb very lightly, letting tension flow out her fingertips.

7 Finish the massage by grasping her hand in yours and raising up her arm. You will not be able to stretch her arm very far at first, but as she grows she'll enjoy the feeling of stretching. All the while, you are also helping to relax your baby/child and to focus her attention on your touch. You are also helping to stimulate blood circulation.

8 Now repeat the same gentle massage as you have just done on the other side, using your left hand this time. What better way to appreciate the fact that the benefits of massage are both emotional and physical.

TIPS FOR PARENTS
1. ARE YOU TALKIN' TO ME?

Talk to your baby. Before you start her massage, tell her what you will be doing and ask her if it is okay. Of course, she won't say, "yes," but she will let you know it's okay by smiling and gurgling. While it's true that a baby will virtually never turn down a massage, make sure you are sensitive to your baby's needs and wants. If she becomes fussy while you're preparing for the massage, or if she squirms with displeasure as you begin, simply stop. You may then try to talk to her and explain again what you would like to do for her. She will understand what you mean by the soothing tone in your voice. If she continues to fuss, simply put off the massage for another time.

Take a minute to think about how you talk to your baby. Parents usually talk to their babies with what is commonly referred to as "baby talk." Basically, baby talk is characterized by a slower cadence, softer tone, and exaggerated inflection of syllables. (And you never knew baby talk was so technical.) The reason we do this is not because it sounds cute (which it does), but rather because it is an instinctive way that we teach our children to speak. By slowing down our speech, and by clearly annunciating each syllable, your child will have a better opportunity to learn her native tongue.

2. SWING YOUR BABY!

Holding both of her hands, stand her up on a table facing you. Tell her you are going to let her hang in the air, and that she will be protected from falling. Then, lift her up off the table just an inch or two. Count to five while you are holding her up, and then ease her back down to the table. Repeat this several times at each massage session, but also re-peat this exercise outside the massage whenever you can. This exercise helps to develop her lungs and chest muscles. You'll be surprised at how straight and strong she will become, and at the rate of her growth.

3. ADD IT UP!

Teach math during your massage. Believe it or not, finger massage is a great time to introduce math. As you massage each finger, start counting one, two, three, four, and five. Say each word distinctly. This really will help your child learn to count. Then do both hands to teach her about addition. Five plus five equals ten!

4. CONGRATULATIONS!

Last, and most important, congratulate your baby and give her a big hug. She's sure to want more of the same loving treatment again soon. Remember that you can never love a baby too much, nor give her too much acknowledgment. Babies love to be loved. Some people think you will spoil a baby if you love them too much. But who among us has ever felt they were loved too much?

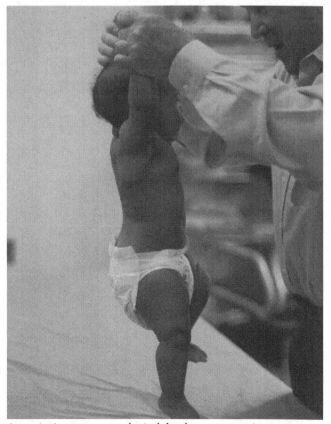

Aya enjoying some neurological development exercises.

HOW TO MASSAGE YOUR CHILD'S CHEST AND SHOULDERS
APPROXIMATE MASSAGE TIME: 5-7 MINUTES

Have your child lie down on his back. Some children prefer to have their knees up. Others down. Allow him to choose—this will let him express his own desires. Stand where you can reach comfortably to his shoulders. Put some oil on your hands, and rub them together to get your hands and the oil warm. Spread the oil gently and evenly across his chest, sides, and shoulders.

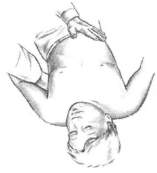

1 Place your right hand just under the left side of his left rib cage, spread your fingers apart, and gently pull the skin and underlying tissue along the ribs as you glide your fingertips down to the side. Flick your fingertips off the side of his body to release any tension.

2 Start moving your palms in a sweeping motion up his chest—the strokes should go vertically up the ribcage and each new stroke should be an inch closer to his side.

3 Repeat steps 1 and 2 on his other side.

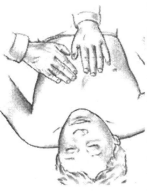

4 Now with one hand on each side of his chest, spread oil up toward her shoulders with your fingertips, working your way up the center of his chest to just below the collarbone. Then inch your way back down the sides of his torso, down to the abdomen, making small circles as you go.

5 Make your way back up his chest, first on the sides until you reach the collarbone, then in the middle. Obviously you are exerting greater pressure with the heel of your hand. Be sure to ask him if he would prefer you to lighten up.

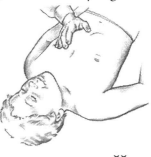

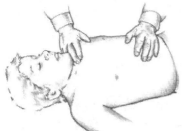

6 Trace the collarbone with your fingers until you reach the left shoulder. Then in a slow, sweeping motion, slide the palm of your hand over the shoulder and down the arm. Do this motion two or three times on each side.

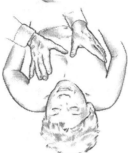

7 Now place a hand, palm down, on each side of his rib cage, thumbs in the middle of the sternum. Use the thumbs to slowly, with minimal pressure, separate his left from right side.

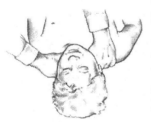

8 Glide both palms up his rib cage, over his shoulders, and cup your hands around either shoulder. Gently squeeze and release the shoulders several times, then take his upper arms in your cupped hands and work down each arm in a milking motion, squeezing out the tension little by little as you move down, and flick the remaining tension out of his fingertips.

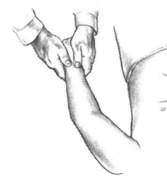

9 Now lightly massage his hand, wrist, and fingers with your fingertips. Place your thumb on top of each hand, fingers underneath her palm, and again sweep the tension out through his fingers.

10 As you finish your massage session, congratulate him for being such a cooperative partner. Remember that you can't praise her enough. He needs your loving encouragement.

TIPS FOR PARENTS

1. STRIKE UP THE BAND!

Expose your child to music. Feel free to play your favorite music or allow him to play his favorite music. (Hopefully it will not be hard rock, because this is the time for a soothing experience.) Besides calming him, and perhaps gently lulling him to sleep, he will begin to experience the wonders of music. That's a legacy that will last a lifetime.

2. TEACH YOUR CHILDREN WELL

Start teaching your child about vital anatomical functions. As you are touching each of his vital areas, especially his heart and lungs, explain their function. Tell him that his body depends upon the oxygen that the lungs deliver to his body and that his entire life force is sustained with each beat of his heart. He's old enough to understand what you are saying, and if you are positive and enthusiastic he will feel the excitement of learning how his body functions.

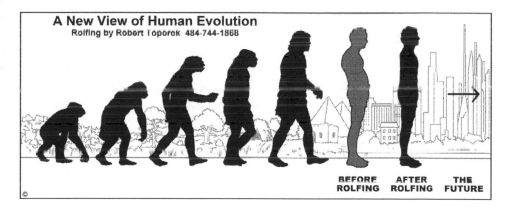

A New View of Human Evolution
Rolfing by Robert Toporek 484-744-1868

BEFORE ROLFING   AFTER ROLFING   THE FUTURE

LEGS AND FEET
OUR STANCE IN LIFE

This little piggy went to market" has been played on countless babies' toes through the ages. You'll probably play it with your baby, and he will enjoy it immensely. What's more, he'll love it when you start massaging his legs and feet.

Standing squarely on your own two feet. Standing up for yourself. Taking a stand. Standing out! These are important expressions that we use to describe various forms of personal strength. They are also statements that relate directly to our legs and feet in a physical and practical manner.

Our legs and feet are essential in developing a sense of wholeness in our bodies and in our lives. When you ask people what they know about their legs and feet, the answers usually address whether they are strong or weak, and how they move. When you ask them how their legs and feet relate to their posture, either in their body or their life, they are often puzzled by the question. Yet people are recognized by their walk and by their stance. No matter how they try to hide it, their posture tells the world something about them.

Our sense of movement in life is directly related to how connected we are to our legs and feet. Maintaining flexibility of the legs and feet is an essential tool in keeping your child prepared to be flexible throughout his life, both physically and emotionally. Some people don't know how to shift their position—some live their entire lives with their foot on the brakes, while others live their lives with their foot on the gas pedal. Flexibility is the key to avoiding these extremes.

Many aspects of formal education are geared toward teaching people how to fit in, as opposed to standing out. This is especially true with children. Children have to learn to get along, follow directions, and suppress their opinions. You know the old saying: "Children should be seen and not heard." Many parents still subscribe to that idea, and some children will go to great lengths to fit in, especially if they do not have a very strong sense of self.

Helping your baby develop her legs and feet—and her stance in life—is one of the most important gifts you can give her. It will give her the self-assurance to face the stresses she'll surely encounter along life's path. This gift will be far more important than any material gift.

Until one is committed there is hesitancy, the chance to draw back, always ineffectiveness.

Concerning all acts of initiative (and creation), there is one elementary truth, the ignorance of which kills countless ideas and splendid plans: that the moment one definitely commits oneself, then Providence moves too.

All sorts of things occur to help one that would never otherwise have occurred.

A whole stream of events issues from the decision, raising in one's favor all manner of unforeseen incidents and meetings and material assistance, which no man could have dreamt would have come his way.

I have learned a deep respect for one of Goethe's couplets: Whatever you dream you can be, begin it. Boldness has genius, power, and magic in it.

–W.H. MURRAY

HOW TO MASSAGE YOUR BABY'S LEGS AND FEET
APPROXIMATE MASSAGE TIME: 5–7 MINUTES

Place your baby on her back with her feet facing you. Put some oil on your hands and rub them together to warm the oil. Spread the oil all over the left foot and leg—both front and back.

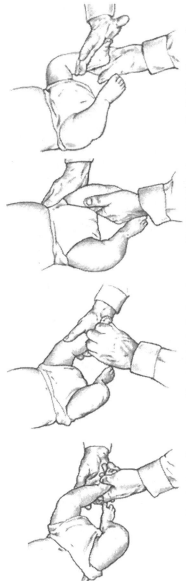

1 With your palm on the top of the left foot, gently brush the leg all the way up to the top of the thigh, applying light pressure as you move slowly and confidently. Brush back down to the foot, and repeat. Then repeat this process for the underside of the leg.

2 Now, starting at your baby's hip, work back down the leg to the foot and ankle by gently squeezing the leg as you rotate it slightly (with your other hand on the foot) in a corkscrew motion to cover all surfaces.

3 Hold her left ankle in your right hand, and with your left hand begin to massage the sole of her foot gently with your thumb. Rub your thumb in a circular motion, from her heel to his toes. Then gently pinch each toe and give it the slightest stretch. Then wiggle your little finger between each toe.

4 Still holding her left foot in your right hand—with your fingers on the bottom and your thumb on top—use a circular motion to gently massage the top of her foot from the ankle area to her toes.

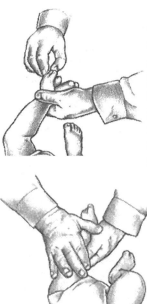

5 This is a great time to start teaching your baby to count. Starting with the big toe, say "one, two, three, four, five" as you touch each toe tip and count aloud. When you are finished, you can work the joints of the feet—just a little—by using your hands to flex the foot and ankle. Push the foot up from the sole with one hand while stabilizing it from underneath with the other. Then, exercise the joint in each toe by very gently tugging on the tip while stabilizing the base of the foot with your free hand.

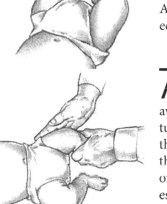

6 Now try stretching the left leg down with one hand while you are stretching up with the other—one hand on top of the leg, the other underneath. Perform this motion ever so gently, working up to the top of the thigh with one hand and down to the ankle with the other. As always, keep your hands relaxed and molded gently to his muscles.

7 Reach up around the hip with your right hand, linger there so that she will become aware of that crucial joint, and then slowly return down the outside of the leg, stroking with the palm of your hand as you go. Carry out this up-and-down motion on the left leg two or three more times (use more oil when necessary).

8 Grasp the calf of her left leg and lift the leg up straight, then alternate between bending the knee and straightening the leg. Try to bring the knee up in a straight line and not out to the side. This helps to lengthen and strengthen the hamstrings.

9 Repeat steps 1 through 8 on the other leg.

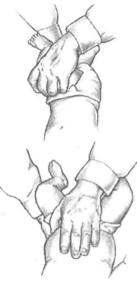

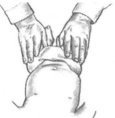

10 Place both of her legs flat on the table. Then, pick up her right leg by the knee and stretch it over across his left leg. This motion stretches all the hip muscles and gets your baby accustomed to using those little legs. Place both legs flat on the table again, and then stretch the left leg over the right.

11 And finally, there's one more step. Reach under your baby's bottom, place your hand flat under the pelvis, palm up, and using your fingertips gently slide your hand out from under her, letting the lower back and pelvis down slowly. In her mind, this motion establishes a connection between massage of the legs and feet with motion of the upper body.

12 Now complete your massage of your baby's legs and feet. With both hands—using very wide brushing motions—brush all of the tension down each leg, into his feet, and out her toes.

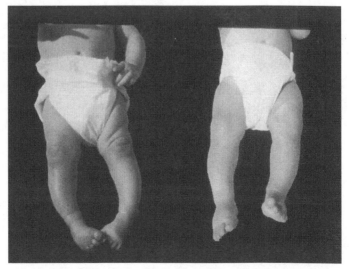

Baby with bowed legs before and after Rolfing by Robert Toporek.

TIPS FOR PARENTS

1. CRAWLING

You want to encourage your baby to crawl, perhaps even earlier than expected. (The key factor here is stimulation—the more stimulation you can provide for her, the faster she will develop.) Place her on the floor face down, with your palms on the soles of her feet. That way she has something to push off on. She may cry or get frustrated—or, with your gentle push, she may take to crawling. Whatever her reaction, early crawling will give her an opportunity to use her legs in conjunction with the rest of her body.

2. LEG STRETCHES

Gently place your baby on her back. Place your fingers underneath her right foot with her heel resting in the crook of your thumb. Now, place your right hand on her right hip for support. Raise her right leg straight up with your hand. As before, you'll be stretching her hamstrings especially, but also all of the muscle groups in her legs. Lower the leg slowly and repeat several times. Always perform this exercise on both legs.

HOW TO MASSAGE YOUR CHILD'S LEGS AND FEET
APPROXIMATE MASSAGE TIME: 10 MINUTES

Place your child on his back, feet toward you. Pour some oil into your hands and rub them together to warm the oil. With your left hand under his left heel to support the foot, gently spread the oil across the top of his left foot, around the ankle, up his calf, over his knee and up his thigh to his pelvis. Then swing your hand underneath his bottom and begin to slide your hand under his leg, then under his knee and calf, down to his ankle. Make sure the oil is distributed evenly around the entire leg.

1 With your right hand, cup his left foot and then gently squeeze his foot down toward the toes, forcing any tension out through the toes.

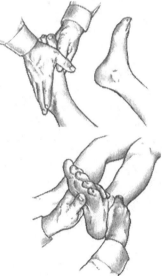

2 Using both thumbs on either side of his left ankle, slowly spread the skin around his ankle from center to side, continuing down his foot toward his toes. Then using the thumb and forefinger of your right hand, gently stretch each toe, both under and on top, then on the sides, lingering for a second at the joints.

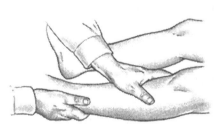

3 With your hand under his left heel, use your thumb to push an imaginary air bubble up to his ankle. Work that bubble up the outside of his calf to the knee. At the knee, take a moment to explore the nooks and crannies under and around the knee with your thumb. Continuing with your thumb, work up his thigh and press that air bubble up as you go. When you reach his hip, place your left hand on the hip and with your right hand, gently stretch the leg down.

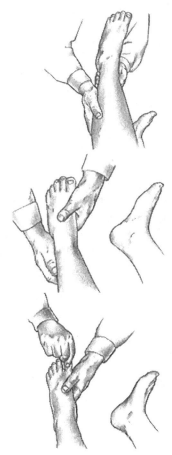

4 Holding his leg up at the thigh with your free hand, bring that air bubble back down again under the thigh with your thumb, then under the calf, and down to the ankle.

5 Use a kneading motion with your forefinger and thumb to massage around his heel.

6 Next, use the heel of your hand to massage around the whole ankle. This part of your hand applies firmer pressure than your previous motions. Work your way back across the top of his foot with the heel of your hand, keeping in mind that this area is more fragile than the ankle—so be aware of how much pressure you are applying.

7 Gently pull each toe, releasing any tension he has built up. Work your way between each toe by rotating your forefinger. If your child is still learning his numbers, count those toes once again, asking your child to count with you.

8 Repeat steps 1 through 7 on his right leg to complete the massage.

TIPS FOR PARENTS

1. BALANCING ACT

Get a flat piece of wood—four inches wide and approximately ten feet long—and place it on the floor. (You can also use tape on the floor to outline such an area.) Encourage your child to practice walking the length of the beam without putting his feet on the floor (or stepping outside the lines). This will be a major step in teaching him balance and poise, two positive developments that will help him stand on his own two feet—both physically and socially. Later, try varying the size of the board. You'll be giving him additional opportunities and challenges as he learns to balance himself.

2. HANGING AROUND

Young children love to hang by their feet. So hold your child's feet by the ankles in both of your hands, turn him upside down, and swing him until he can't stop giggling. Gently lower him back to the floor, asking him if he wants to be swung again. Nine times out of ten the answer is an emphatic, "Yes!"

"Balance in our bodies–our bodies' relationship to gravity–is reflected in behavior states since self expression is intimately related to muscular tone. Balance is a resting state–a capacity and preparedness to respond depending on the stimulus. Imbalance, then, is the movement or impulse to move which when it completes itself, returns to balance. However, many responses never do complete themselves, therefore our bodies and lives remain in what is called habits and patterns. Massage/Rolfing a child can help clear their accumulated tensions and allow your babies/children to live more fully in the present."

DR. IDA ROLF/ROBERT TOPOREK

SIDES OF THE BODY
THE MANY SIDES OF LIFE

Your child grows at a faster rate just after birth than she will at any other time in her life. Savor each moment, for rapid changes will occur before your very eyes. As Bob Dylan once sang: "The times, they are a changin'." We all have attitudes and positions in regard to change. These attitudes and positions are rooted in our bodies. Look at your child from the side and determine whether she is open and flexible or rigid and stiff. Looking at your child sideways will tell you much about her attitude, self-esteem, and ability to embrace change. A child who stands upright will appear more flexible and prepared to react than a child who is slouched over. The more open and flexible she is with her body, the more flexible she will be in all aspects of her life.

As people age, many often subscribe to the maxim that you can't teach an old dog new tricks. Why do so many people resist change? This may be due to the fact that they see things only as "black and white"—with no room for compromise. Or they see the glass as half empty instead of half full, and feel that nothing can be done about it. Yet change is multidimensional; it includes nurturing old attitudes and beliefs that are positive, cutting away old ideas that have proved invalid, and embracing new ideas and situations as they are presented. In short, creating room for change means being flexible.

Those who cannot accept change can be spotted easily—their bodies are rigid and unyielding, so stuck in one position that they do not have the ability to change physically (or otherwise). Many people who experience this inability to seek and embrace change are actually proud of their set ways. They never realize that their thoughts and behavior affect their posture, and vice versa. Yet if their bodies could become more flexible, their ability to change other aspects of their lives could also be improved dramatically. This mind–body connection is the basis for the importance of massage. When someone is willing to change, the results can be quite remarkable.

As far as your baby is concerned, your own flexibility—or lack there-of—can make a dramatic difference in her development. She can become outgoing, accepting of others, and able to deal with different situations, or she can become uptight, rigid, and withdrawn. You can make the choice! You can make the difference!

One of the best ways of helping your child deal with her periods of change is through massage. By working with her body, you can help her handle negative experiences and present her with new options for approaching the inevitable changes in her life and in her body. Moreover, the best way of monitoring her physical and emotional development is through watching her postural changes.

Our children will spend most of their lives in the twenty-first century—a century that will be filled with unprecedented changes! Who we are as parents, families, neighbors, and citizens will change dramatically. One of the most powerful ways you can prepare your child for these changes is by keeping her body flexible—her flexibility in all other areas of life will follow.

Another important ingredient in regard to change and flexibility is communication. Communication makes the world go around, and the more communication skills you give your child, the more world she will have to experience. Give your child ample math knowledge and the physical world will be easier for her to understand. As her reading skills increase, the world of ideas will open up to her. And the more she is massaged, the more comfortable she will become with touch—another vital form of communication.

Each age brings with it the exploration of new behaviors and the testing of new limits. We often fail to keep up with our children's growth and development. Begin to look at your own willingness to change and grow with your child. Most parents try to get children to fit into their world and their lives rather than trying to fit into their child's world. But communication with your child should be a two-way street—for all the lessons you will try to impart, you must always be accepting of the wisdom your child may offer, too.

Because massage will become a family activity, it will also allow your child to accept more readily the changes that occur within the family experience—the loss of relatives, illnesses, moving, starting a new school, and so forth. All of these changes put additional stress on our children. Massage is a great way of dealing with those stresses.

HOW TO MASSAGE YOUR BABY'S SIDES
APPROXIMATE MASSAGE TIME: 7–10 MINUTES

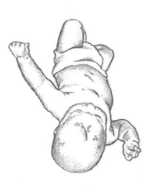

1 Put some oil on your hands and rub them together briskly to warm the oil. Lay your baby on her right side and place a pillow against her back so she won't fall over. Stand beside her.

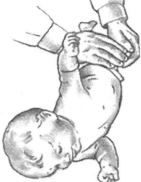

2 With her right leg straight, bring her left leg over the right leg by bending her knee slightly. Place your hand on the inside of her left thigh to stabilize it. Starting at her left knee, use your right hand to spread the oil along the front and outside of her thigh. Use the palm of your hand to massage up to and around her hip using a slow, steady, upward stroke.

3 Slide your hand back down to her knee in one motion along the outside of her thigh, lightly sweeping away the tension as your hand flicks off her skin.

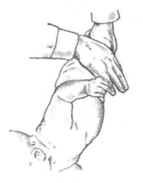

4 Place your right thumb just above the knee on the side of the leg. Picture a line going up the outside of her thigh from the knee to the hip—this is the midline. In a spreading motion, work your thumb from this midline point to the outside of her thigh, then return to the midline and repeat the spreading motion—midline to outside—as you move up to her hip. Return to the knee and repeat the exercise.

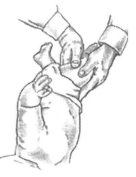

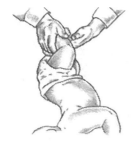

5 Put some more oil on your hands and warm it. Place your palm on her left heel and spread the oil up the back and side of the calf toward the knee. Use a long sweeping motion to come back down to the heel, lightly working the tension down and out of her body. Then locate the midline of her leg at the top of her ankle, and with your thumb work back up her leg—in a spreading motion—from the midline to the outside of her calf.

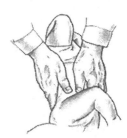

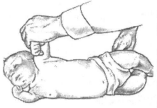

6 Put more oil on your hands and warm it. Apply the oil up along her ribcage to her armpit using long, sweeping motions.

7 Picture the midline running up the side of her torso from the hip to the armpit. Apply firm pressure with your fingertips as you stroke down off the side of the torso, moving up toward the armpit with each new stroke.

8 For the finishing touch of this massage, while she is still lying on her right side, lift her left arm and stretch it up over her head in a straight line toward the ceiling. This gentle stretching motion will emphasize her entire side.

9 Repeat steps 1 through 8 on the other side.

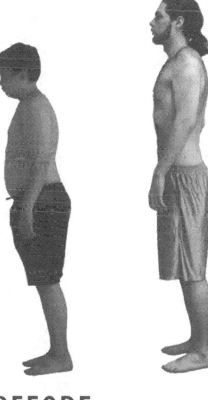

BEFORE   AFTER

Justin before and after Rolfing over six years.

TIPS FOR PARENTS

1. OPPOSITES

Start by getting a warm cloth and a cloth that has been rinsed in cold water. When you touch her arm with the warm cloth, say the word "warm." Then touch her arm on the same spot with the cold cloth, and say "cold." You are creating distinctions, which lead to change. She'll encounter situations demanding change throughout life, and your early training with opposites will help her understand change. Repeat the "opposites" game with a smooth piece of material such as silk or nylon and then with a rough piece of material such as wool, saying the words "smooth" and "rough."

2. START WITH YOURSELF

Change is the law of the land. Nature is always changing. Many human beings, however, are creatures of habit and resist change. They do the same thing the same way, over and over, whether or not it is working. One of my mantras is "In life we have two choices—to grow or shrink. "

Ever notice how the past persists unless interrupted?

Each year, I review my life and ask myself how I can grow or move in a new direction. Sometimes it's in the realm of communication, other times it's in how I dress, or oftentimes I like to just turn my life upside down. This book and program will, at seventy years of age, give me a whole new phase of growth. It has already put me in touch with people and places I never dreamed of.

People all too often stay stuck in the same patterns because change, by its very nature, creates upset. And upset, while not always bad, interrupts the status quo. So it comes as no surprise that parents often try to keep their children "in a box."

Massaging your baby or child on a regular basis alone will change your ideas about child-rearing and allow you to grow with them.

HOW TO MASSAGE YOUR CHILD'S SIDES
APPROXIMATE MASSAGE TIME: 7–10 MINUTES

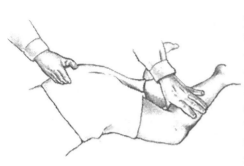

1 Lay your child on a comfortable table or bed on his right side with his head facing away from you. Stand by the side of the bed or table so that you are positioned just below his waistline. Bend his left knee across the bed so that leg is supporting him. Put some oil on your hands and rub them together to warm it. Spread the oil up along the outside of his midline (the midline runs vertically up the side of his ribcage) to just under her arm. Then spread the oil across the inside of the midline (toward his stomach), working back down to the waist.

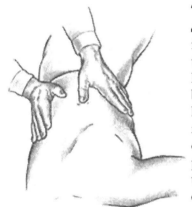

2 Place your right hand on his side just above the hip. Place your left hand on the front of the ribcage to stabilize him during the massage. (Let your supporting hand follow your working hand as it moves up the body.) Using the palm and heel of your right hand, work up his side with small circular motions—start from the hip and concentrate on the outside of the midline, applying firm pressure along the ribs, moving up to under the arm. Now come back down on the inside of the midline, using the same circular motions. Repeat.

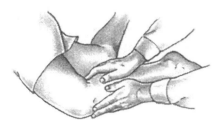

3 Put some more oil on your hands, warm it, and spread the oil up along the midline of the leg from the heel all the way up to the hip. Be sure to cover both sides of the midline.

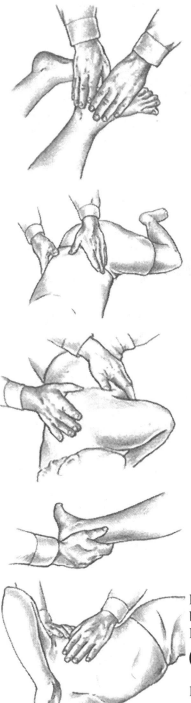

4 With your right hand on the midline at his ankle, start moving your fingertips up his leg in circular motions, always moving from the midline to the outside of his leg, and up to the knee. Continue from the knee and massage up to the hip using circular motions from the midline to the outside of the leg. Switch hands and repeat this motion on the inside of his midline from the ankle to the hip.

5 Next you are going to use your thumbs. Begin at his waist and trace the top of the pelvic bone from the midline toward the center of his lower back. Repeat with slightly more pressure.

6 Then go back to the pelvis and, applying slight pressure with your right thumb, move on up his side—using diagonal strokes from the midline out—until you reach his shoulder. Trace each rib with your thumb and finish each stroke by sweeping your thumb off her back. Continue until you have reached under his arm. Remember to use your opposite hand for support. Change hands and repeat this procedure along the inside of his ribcage.

7 Now move down to the ankle. Using your right thumb, slowly massage up his leg to the knee using small diagonal strokes from the midline out. Continue up the leg until you have reached the pelvis. Switch hands and repeat this procedure on the inside of the midline.

8 Finally, place your palm on the midline under his arm and swiftly sweep your hand down along the midline and off his body at the ankle. Give the ankle and foot a little squeeze at the end of the session.

9 Repeat steps 1 through 8 on his other side. At the end of the complete session, give him a big hug and congratulate him on a great massage!

TIPS FOR PARENTS

1. PLAY THE CHANGE GAME

Children tend to get very engrossed in what they are doing and don't know when to stop. Because of this, they often think they don't have to listen. If they are on a certain track and refuse to be interrupted, one of the best ways of handling this situation is to turn listening into a game.

Get your child's attention and tell her you are going to play a game. But instead of "Simon says," make it "Mommy or Daddy says." Ask your child to put her left hand up and then down, then her right hand up and then down. Have him reach down and touch the floor. Have him stand up. Have him drop his head back and straighten up. Once he is completely engrossed in this game, you might ask him what he was so absorbed in before the game, and ask him how he came to switch gears. He will have broken a pattern and accepted the reality of change. You can vary this game in many different ways.

2. STOP-START GAME

Tell your child you are going to play "stop-start." Get a coloring book and some crayons and ask him to start coloring until you say "stop." Then he must stop immediately. Create a reward system for him stopping right away. Again let him color, then say "stop." You can add different elements to this game. For instance, have him run around the room, stopping the instant you tell him to stop. This exercise causes him to listen and to integrate his body with starting and stopping. But to your child, this is also a fun game to play with Mommy or Daddy.

INNER LEGS
VITALITY

Vitality is a quality that is expressed through the way we stand, walk, and move. Happy children love to run, skip, jump, explore, tussle, play, dance, sing, and turn everything into a game. In short, they love to live life. Massaging your child's inner legs and pelvic area can make a big difference in his vitality—helping him develop vital tendencies and encouraging him to maintain this vitality for a lifetime.

So what happens as we become adults? The older we get, the more we blame our lack of vitality on aging. Traditionally, becoming a grown-up is to become stiffer and tighter with each passing year until, by the time we are forty or fifty, our bodies begin to sag more noticeably and the aches and pains increase. You can notice this lack of vitality in your walk and in your posture. We have been taught that life is hard and serious, but by maintaining a strong sense of vitality we can keep it light and lively. Wouldn't it be great to grow up and to keep our zest for life?

Young children, unfortunately, often have to grow up in an adult world with tired and achy parents and with teachers who have been conditioned to keep their emotions in check. Once your child starts preschool or school, make it a point to spend time in his classroom—this is one of the ways you can monitor what he is learning about vitality from the influences that surround him. One of the things you will find quite striking is how kids move around the classroom. Happy children usually skip or trot everywhere they can. Others may slouch around or move more slowly. Be sure to notice how your child moves around the classroom.

Vitality plays a major part in many aspects of your child's development. How vital is he in approaching homework? What level of vitality does he exude when he expresses himself in a group? How energetic is he while at play? Obviously, you want to raise a lively child who is not afraid to express himself in words and in actions.

Another part of life that relates to the inside of the legs and pelvis is sexuality. This is closely linked to our overall vitality because, as sexual beings, the act of sexual love invigorates us mentally and physically.

As our culture becomes more open to publicly discussing or displaying sexuality, children are bombarded with mixed messages: "Have sex." "Don't have sex." "Boast about your sexual experiences." "Don't talk about your sexual experiences."

By massaging the area of your child's pelvis and inner thighs, you can give him a better sense of his body and a better understanding of and control over his sexual life. You must, however, respect any embarrassment he feels concerning these areas. Be very gentle and communicative when you massage this sensitive area. You do not need to touch the groin area, but be sure not to exaggerate your avoidance of the area. If your child expresses discomfort, simply move on.

You can create an environment in your family of openness and communication. Thus, you can help him better understand the changes his body will go through, create for him a very healthy attitude about his sexuality, and ensure that his level of vitality will remain high.

HOW TO MASSAGE YOUR BABY'S INNER LEGS
APPROXIMATE MASSAGE TIME: 5–7 MINUTES

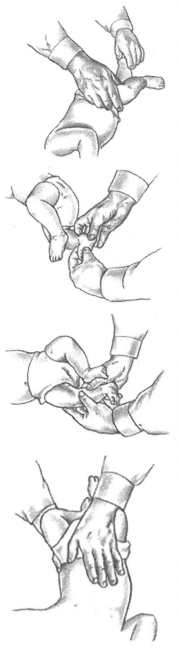

1 Place your baby on her right side, with her feet facing you and a pillow behind his back to give her support. Bend her left knee up toward her chest so that it leaves the inside of her right leg unobstructed. Rub some oil on your hands to warm it up. With your right hand at the top of her right pelvic bone, use a light brushing motion to spread the oil over the inside of her leg, making sure to cover the entire leg including the foot.

2 Cup your hands and place them under her right foot. With the thumbs of both hands under her middle toe, move your thumbs in a circular spreading motion across the sole of her foot, over her heel, and up to the ankle. Repeat.

3 Visualize an imaginary midline along the side of her leg (where the seam of a pair of pants runs) and place your thumbs on this midline at the ankle. Starting with both thumbs on this midline, begin to spread your thumbs away from the midline—one going left and one going right. Do this all the way up the leg—over the calf, knee, and thigh—stopping as close to the rim of her pelvis as you can get. Then work back down the leg to the ankle using the same spreading motion with your thumbs. Repeat this motion up and down her leg two or three times.

4 Turn your baby over and repeat steps 1 through 3 on the other leg.

5 Turn your baby on her back, place your fingers under her pelvis with your thumbs on top of the pelvic bone, and gently pull down to lengthen the spine. Give her a big hug and thank him for a great massage!

TIPS FOR PARENTS

1. BICYCLE KICKS

The bicycling exercise you probably learned as a child is really great for giving your baby exercise as well as generating enthusiasm. Lay her on her back and raise her knees to her chest. Take a foot in each hand and begin moving her legs in a cycling fashion. Vary the speed of your revolutions and, as you do, announce the different speeds you're applying. Go slow, then moderate speed, then fast, and repeat each speed a couple of times. She'll probably reward you with a big smile because she'll be having fun. And you'll be stimulating her both physically and mentally. Give her a big hug. (Always remember that you can't hug a baby too much.)

2. SWING YOUR BABY!

Babies love to swing. Hold your baby under the arms and gently swing her round and round. Then hold her by the feet and carefully swing her upside down. Swinging your baby helps her brain deal with balance by creating what is known as "vestibular stimulation"—you're stimulating the part of the brain that deals with balance. And if your child tends to get hyper, this swinging motion can help bring her back into balance.

3. BABY BOUNCE

Babies also love to be bounced up in the air. Bounce your baby lightly in the air, never really letting your hands release from her body. The thrill of whirling up into the air exhilarates almost all babies. As you progress you can bounce her higher and higher, just as long as you assure her that you won't let her fall.

HOW TO MASSAGE YOUR CHILD'S INNER LEGS
APPROXIMATE MASSAGE TIME: 7–10 MINUTES

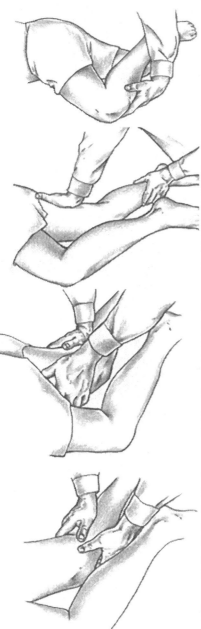

1 Lay your child on his right side, facing away from you. Bend his left leg up and over his right leg—letting the left leg lie stretched out on the bed so that you can work on his right leg. Put oil on your hands and rub them together to warm the oil. Spread the oil up the inside or your child's right leg from the knee up to the edge of his pelvis.

2 Visualize the midline of his right inner leg (like where the seam of a pair of pants runs). Using the heel of your right hand, begin to work the tension out of your toddler's thigh using light sweeping motions from the midline toward the back of the leg. Start at the knee and move each stroke higher until you reach the pelvis.

3 Now use the heel of your left hand. Starting at the midline above the knee, apply short sweeping strokes from the midline to the front of the leg. Move each stroke farther up until you reach the pelvis.

4 Repeat steps 2 and 3—right hand toward the back of the leg, left toward the front of the leg—two or three times on the upper part of the leg.

5 Rub more oil on your hands and place both thumbs on the midline at the knee (the inside point of the knee). Use your right fingers and thumb to trace the back and right sides of the knee; use your left thumb and fingers to trace the top and left sides of the knee. Explore the contours of the knee with your thumbs and fingertips.

6 Apply more oil to your hands and rub them together. Apply a liberal, even coating of oil to the knee, calf, ankle, and foot.

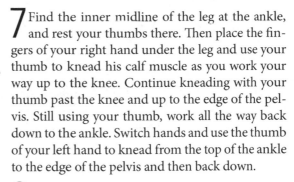

7 Find the inner midline of the leg at the ankle, and rest your thumbs there. Then place the fingers of your right hand under the leg and use your thumb to knead his calf muscle as you work your way up to the knee. Continue kneading with your thumb past the knee and up to the edge of the pelvis. Still using your thumb, work all the way back down to the ankle. Switch hands and use the thumb of your left hand to knead from the top of the ankle to the edge of the pelvis and then back down.

8 Next use your right hand to erase the midline and create the idea of a whole leg. Do this by using a circular motion. Start at the top of the leg and move all the way down to the ankle, creating small circles that go from the back of the leg to the front. Repeat this two or three times. When you reach the ankle, push more tension away.

9 Next, squeeze, caress, wiggle, massage, and explore the contours of the foot. Alternate your hands on different parts of the foot and explore using different motions to take all the tension out of your child's toes and feet.

Remember to massage each toe and make sure that you massage between each toe.

10 To finish, put a little more oil on your hands and, alternating between your left and right hands, start at the top of the leg and sweep down the leg in one long vertical motion, bringing all the tension out of the entire leg. Use your palms to apply medium pressure, and repeat the stroke twice with each hand. Then use your fingers—in short sweeping strokes that move from the mid line in or out—to go from the top of the leg to the ankle and foot. At the end give his foot a little squeeze.

11 Repeat steps 1 through 10 with him lying on his left side. When you are through, give him a big hug and congratulate him on a really great massage.

TIPS FOR PARENTS

1. HAMSTRING STRETCH

Hamstrings are the large muscles on the back of the thigh. They often get tight and need to be stretched. You can establish a simple hamstring stretch that will help your child reap benefits throughout his life.

Put your child on his back and bend his knees so they are at a 45-degree angle. Put one hand on each knee and, alternately, slowly push each knee toward his chest until you feel some resistance. Push gently past the resistance—just a little bit. This stretches the important hamstring muscles and will leave your toddler feeling fit and energized.

2. RUNNING

Running is a great way to build up your toddler's energy and vitality. Run with him in short bursts, going as fast as you can for twenty yards or so, and then walk a short distance, and then run again. You can turn this running exercise into a game—take turns shouting out "Walk!" or "Run!" Encourage your toddler to have as much fun as possible.

Toddlers love to make noise, so encourage him to whoop and holler while he's running. You can whoop and holler too!

"There are only two lasting bequeaths we can hope to give our children. One of these is roots, the other wings."

JOHANN WOLFGANG VON GOETHE

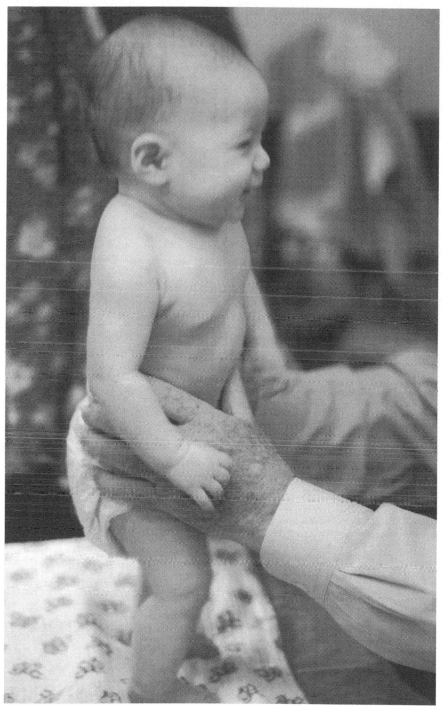

Three-month-old baby after ten Rolfing sessions.

ABDOMEN
POWER AND CONFIDENCE

Mongolian warriors have long been considered some of the most fearless warriors of all time. Their bravery is believed to stem in part from the fact that before and after each battle they would spend a complete day performing self-massage. These massages were a ritual in which they massaged away any fear they had accumulated before and after each battle.

It could be said that human beings, by nature, are afraid and defensive. This can be explained in purely physical terms: the flexor muscles generally overpower the extensor muscles. In other words, the body often tenses up naturally and unconsciously (flexors) more than it tends to relax (extensors). This pattern begins the instant a baby comes out of the womb. Massage can help counteract this ingrained pattern, and gradually the action of the extensor muscles will become balanced with that of the flexor muscles. The result is that one is able to overcome tension by conditioning the body to be more relaxed. The more relaxed one is, the more powerful one can be.

Many people react to challenges by first tensing up their stomach. We often call this tense feeling "butterflies." You also hear people commenting about rough situations by saying that they have "a pit in their stomach." Massage is a very useful tool in relieving and preventing these natural adversaries.

In order to successfully massage your child's abdomen and impart the feeling of power, you have to examine your own attitude toward upsets. If you spend considerable time being upset, you need to adopt a new attitude in which power and confidence will overcome those upsets.

You've heard the expression "Don't sweat the small stuff." That's a good philosophy to adopt and to pass on to your children. Of course, it's necessary to teach them about the dangers in life's path that they should avoid, but you should also teach them to avoid unnecessary anxiety concerning minor stresses and inconveniences.

It is harmful to continually tell a child not to touch something "because you'll break it," or to always say, "Don't run because you'll hurt yourself."

It's up to you to distinguish between real danger and the unrealistic fears that may be of your own making. It is of utmost importance to teach children not to let their fears immobilize them.

Children need a certain freedom and latitude to make discoveries for themselves, to try new things and to take chances. Children manage to accumulate many scrapes and cuts in their day, but their wounds can be tended to easily without wounding their psyches. In fact, patching up a wound is a good time to "kiss it and make it better." You'll be bonding with your child in the process, and they'll learn that they can overcome upsets.

Generally, children are taught to fear upsets. We say to them, "If you're going to get upset, take a time-out or go to your room." What is the message we're giving in this instance? It is one of reprimand, and that's not always good! Imagine teaching your child how to experience a powerful, constructive upset. Or, even better, how to solve a big upset. Powerful people are able to resolve upsets because they have a good attitude toward dealing with upsets. Mostly they are confident that they can overcome the upset, and that confidence alone can be the catalyst for overcoming the upset.

It's not easy to develop a powerful, confident child. However, by massaging a child's abdomen, you can help alleviate his fears and assist him in expressing any upsets he may be holding in.

Being powerful is different from being forceful. Many people discourage their children from being too powerful for fear that the child will be perceived as forceful or obnoxious. Allowing your child to experience healthy power and confidence will pay off in huge dividends later on in life.

HOW TO MASSAGE YOUR BABY'S ABDOMEN
APPROXIMATE MASSAGE TIME: 3 MINUTES

1 Start by laying your baby on her back, feet toward you. Place oil on your hands and make sure the oil is warm. Apply an even layer of oil along the pelvis, up the sides of the ribcage, and over the entire stomach and chest area.

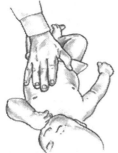

2 Place your right hand palm-down in the middle of her chest, and hold your hand there for several seconds to feel her breathing pattern. Using the outside of your hand, trace the edge of her rib cage from the center to her left side. Repeat two or three times. Then follow the same motion with your left hand, tracing her rib cage from the center of her chest out to her right side.

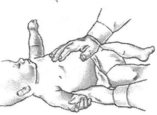

3 Place your left hand under her back for support and, with your right hand just below her waist, use a brushing motion to lightly spread oil from the center of the abdomen out to the sides—one side at a time. Be careful around her belly button because this is an especially sensitive area for newborns. Work down to her pelvic area with gentle strokes—starting from the midline of the abdomen and finishing at the pelvic bone. As each stroke ends, feel your hands sweeping tension down and out of your child's sides. Make sure you pay equal attention to both sides.

4 Next place both hands under her back at midspine and gently glide your fingers down the back, stretching the skin and muscle from her spine to either side as you go. Repeat the stretching motion, from the spine to each of her sides, two or three times.

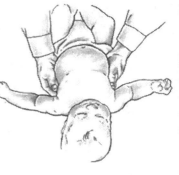

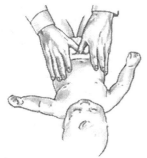

5 With the fingers of your right hand, work back down the front of her body from below the rib cage to the pelvic area, drawing little circles around her abdomen clockwise. Repeat with your left hand. Then with the palm of each hand, gently sweep the tension out of her sides again in broad, light strokes. In very young babies, this massage should take two to three minutes. Increase the time as your baby gets older.

TIPS FOR PARENTS

1. SIT-UPS

A very young baby may seem too fragile to participate in strength-training exercises, but that's not the case. A good and safe exercise for a baby (or for anyone!) is the sit-up, which helps develop and strengthen the abdominal and back muscles.

Place your baby on her back with his knees bent and feet flat. Stand over her and take her wrists in your hands. Gently pull her up to a sitting position. Then lower him, also very gently. Be sure to tell her what you are doing and how it is going to strengthen her abdomen and lower back. Repeat the sit-up two or three times at first. Soon you'll feel her growing stronger and straighter, at which time you can increase the number of sit-ups at each session. Be sure to do this exercise with fun and enthusiasm, and she'll soon learn that exercise is fun as well as rewarding.

2. ROLLING ON A BEACH BALL

Buy a big beach ball at a toy store. She'll love it from the start with its bright colors, and she'll love it even more when you tell her how much fun you are going to have together with the ball. Place her stomach-down on the ball, with your hand on her back for support. Then roll her around on top of the ball. She'll probably be squealing with delight as she is rolled back and forth several times. In the process, her abdominal muscles will be developing and strengthening, clearly establishing the foundation for future development of power and confidence that comes with strength and self-assurance.

HOW TO MASSAGE YOUR CHILD'S ABDOMEN

APPROXIMATE MASSAGE TIME: 5 MINUTES

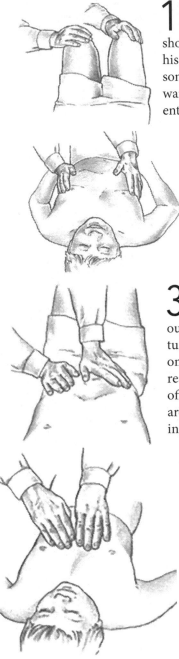

1 Lay your child on his back and bend his knees up to give his lower back extra support. His feet should be flat on the bed or table. Stand or sit by his feet with his head pointing away from you. Put some oil on your hands and rub them together to warm the oil and your hands. Apply the oil to his entire abdomen, sides, pelvic area, and lower chest.

2 Place the heels of your palms on his lower abdomen, and let your fingertips rest on his rib cage. Allow your hands to rest there until you feel his abdomen relax. Begin moving the heel of your hands straight up toward the rib cage until you reach the first rib. Let your hands separate and work toward either side with a very light brushing motion; brush the tension out of his sides.

3 Place the palms of each hand on the middle of the sternum. Now begin to sweep your palms out to the sides. Work down his abdomen by returning your palms to a slightly lower position on the midline after each stroke until you have reached the top of the pelvis. As each stroke lifts off the side of your child's body, imagine that you are drawing the tension out of his body and flicking it away.

4 Next you'll be raking the abdomen with your fingertips using short, firm motions. Starting at the sternum, and working down his body as above, use the fingertips of each hand to rake the tension out of your child's abdomen. You'll begin to feel the abdominal wall stretch slightly as you rake down. Don't put too much pressure on the downward motion at first, but rather start off raking lightly. As you get more comfortable with this motion you can begin to go deeper. Always gauge your child's pressure by his reaction, and by questioning him as to how he feels.

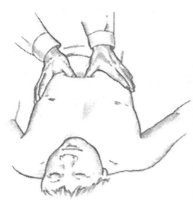

5 Finally you want to stretch the abdomen. This move has lots of variations, so feel free to be creative once you have learned the basic motions. Begin by placing the thumbs of each hand together on the center of the sternum. Then use your thumbs to trace the bottom of the rib cage out toward the sides and down toward the back.

At the end of this motion return to the abdomen. Now place your thumbs at the midline of his torso just below the rib cage and start stretching the abdomen out toward the sides. Return your thumbs to the center of the abdomen after each stroke, moving them down slightly each time. Continue this stretching motion until you reach the edge of his pelvis, then work back up to the waist again. You'll be pulling lots of accumulated tension out of his body.

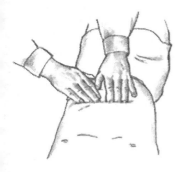

6 Rub a little more oil into your hands. Place your fingertips just below the rib cage and trace firm circles all the way down to the top of his pelvic bone. Do this two or three times, moving your hands apart toward the sides as you go.

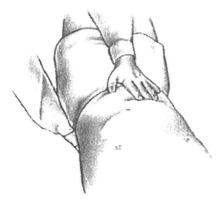

7 To bring this session to an end, place your hands on either side of the rib cage. Slowly and lightly begin to sweep all the excess tension down and out of his belly. Do this two or three times and then congratulate your child for successfully completing another exceptional massage.

TIPS FOR PARENTS

1. LIFTING WEIGHTS

Many parents wouldn't think of letting their small children work out with weights, even though they appreciate the need for children to grow strong. When you buy light weights (starting with half-pound weights and working up to two pound weights) and let him begin to lift them with his hands, he'll be gaining confidence as well as strength. Nothing instills confidence as much as having a fit body.

2. ENCOURAGE UPSETS

Sometimes kids will stage an upset as a tool to manipulate their parents. They do this because they think it will intimidate. Instead of becoming intimidated, let your child learn that it's okay to get upset. And let him fully express why he is upset. Help him discover that an upset is a prelude to communication—it doesn't necessarily mean he should get what he wants. Also teach him your limits in terms of upsets. He can only go so far before you discipline him. You'll have a more cooperative child, and he will gain respect for your standards.

"God put us here to prepare this place for the next generation. That's our job. Raising children and helping the community, that's preparing for the next generation."

DIKEMBE MUTOMBO

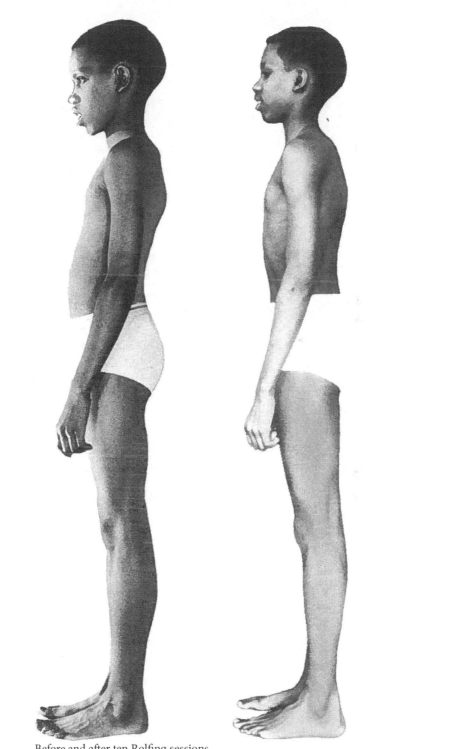

Before and after ten Rolfing sessions.

EXTENSOR MUSCLES
EXTENDING YOURSELF

All along the back of your legs, your buttocks, and your back are muscles called "extensors." These extensors are an important group of muscles that enable us to fully extend ourselves. They help keep our bodies in good shape, control our posture, and also help maintain good energy flow. Extensors are often at odds with an opposite group of muscles called "flexors," which are the muscles responsible for contraction. Typically, the flexor muscles overpower the extensors. A good example of this is the fetal position babies take on in the womb. After birth they begin to straighten out, and a regular massage program is a great way to facilitate this process.

In psychological terms, humanity, one might say, has not yet fully extended itself. Many of us are still living with—and inadvertently passing on to our children—old patterns of constriction and fear that restrict us both physically and emotionally.

Restrictive patterns are continuously reinforced through cultural conditioning. When most people think of "extending themselves," they usually think in terms of taking on more responsibility or more burdens. We all learn in one way or another not to extend ourselves too far. (Consider how rarely people choose to "go out on a limb.") When we do, we feel we become too vulnerable and are liable to get hurt. This applies to both physical and emotional situations.

Moreover, when our ideas or beliefs are rejected, we often perceive this as a rejection of ourselves. This is especially true among children. Children can sometimes be brutally honest, not very nice, or even downright mean and nasty to each other. Incidents in which one is rejected in some way train us to stay cool, reserved, protected, and invulnerable. No matter how much you do to protect your children, however, they will still have to learn to live in a bigger world which may not be as kind and gentle as you are.

As Henry Miller once said, "If you have the vision and the urge to undertake great tasks, then you will discover in yourself the virtues and capabilities required for their accomplishments. Perhaps only when you have come to the end of your resources will the light dawn. It is only when we admit our limitations that we find there are no limitations."

Accomplished people no doubt understand the importance of extending themselves to others and to their projects. They also know that pain and setbacks are simply obstructions on the road to achievement. For example, Walt Disney failed many times before Disneyland was successful. Abraham Lincoln failed to win elections to various offices before he was finally elected President. There are countless cases of people who have gone beyond their limits to discover new territory for themselves and others. Extending themselves was vital to their success.

It is important to continue to live fully—constantly expanding and stretching your capabilities—and to encourage and empower your children to do the same. You can enable your children to break the grip of fear while you teach them how to use their extensor muscles to extend themselves physically and otherwise. Massage is a great way of helping your baby and child strengthen the extensor muscles and begin to learn how to use them in ways that will result in power and confidence.

HOW TO MASSAGE YOUR BABY'S EXTENSOR MUSCLES
APPROXIMATE MASSAGE TIME: 8 MINUTES

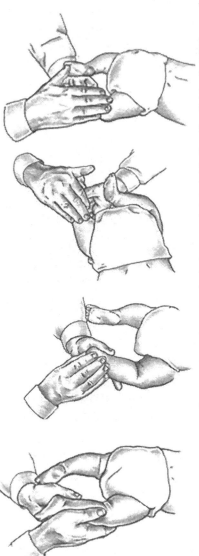

1 Lay your baby down on her stomach. Position yourself at the bottom of her feet. Apply oil to your hands and rub them together briskly to warm the oil, and spread it all the way up the back of her right leg. Make sure you cover the entire back of the leg, as well as the sides and the foot.

2 Squeeze her tiny calf muscles. Caress the tender area behind the knee. When you reach the top of the leg, use your fingertips to lightly rake down the entire leg. Hand over hand, let your fingers run lightly from the top to the bottom of the back of her leg.

3 Take her right foot and hold it in your left hand. Use your fingertips to stimulate the bottom of her foot—her heel, insole, and the ball of her foot.

Feel the texture of her skin, her crinkles and wrinkles. Pay special attention to her toes—massage each one, making sure you get in between each toe as well.

4 Now wrap both of your hands around her right leg just above the ankle, making sure your palms are against the back part of the leg. Using a slow rope-climbing motion, hand over hand, massage up the front of her leg.

5 Repeat steps 1 through 4 on her left leg.

6 Apply more oil to your hands and return your attention to her right leg. Place both your thumbs together in the center of the back of her leg, just above the ankle. Using a kneading motion, spread the oil out to either side. With a light pressure, let your thumbs massage her leg as if you were kneading a lump of dough. Do this all the way up the entire leg until you reach the buttocks, always working from the center outward.

7 Oil your hands and repeat step 6 on the left leg.

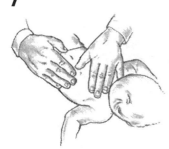

8 Now stand on the left side of your baby's body. Spread oil across her entire back from the buttocks to the shoulders. Use your palm and fingertips to gently stroke up along the left side of her back up to the shoulder and then down the right side to the waist—really feel the muscles as you go. Then, reverse your direction, moving up the right side, across the shoulders and spine, and down the left side.

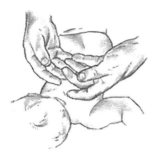

9 Now use the fronts of your fingers (both hands) to massage her back. Move your fingers in a crisscross motion up and down the sides of the spine. Let the skin slide between your fingers as you go. When you reach the top of the shoulders, fan your fingers out to the sides and across the shoulder blades. Then bring your hands together in the center of the spine at the nape of the neck and follow the spine down the middle of the back.

10 Place your fingertips at the nape of the neck, lightly brush down her back and legs, and force all the tension out of her body.

11 Now turn your baby over so that she is lying on her back with her knees up and feet flat. Raise her pelvis up gently and position your right hand, palm up, on her tailbone right above her buttocks. Place your left hand on the front of the torso, right below the rib cage. Now with your right hand begin to lightly stretch the lower muscles of her back by gently pulling down on the area two to three inches above the tail bone, applying slight pressure with the left hand. Then gently ease her down flat.

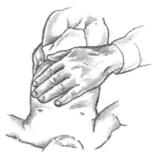

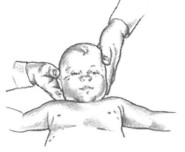

12 Now reposition yourself behind your baby with her head facing you. Cradle the back of her neck with both of your hands. Gently move your hands up and down either side of her neck, lightly pulling on the muscles as you move, lengthening the spine.

TIPS FOR PARENTS
1. STRETCH YOUR BABY

First, lay your baby comfortably on her back. Take her right hand and bring it across the body to touch the left shoulder. Then reverse, taking the left hand across the body to the right shoulder. Next, place the heel of her right leg in your hand and slowly raise the leg up, stretching the hamstrings. Then switch legs, taking hold of the left heel and slowly raising the leg. Now bend her knees so the soles of her feet are flat on the table. Gently rock the knees from side to side to loosen up the hip joints.

"I have learned that raising children is the single most difficult thing in the world to do. It takes hard work, love, luck, and a lot of energy, and it is the most rewarding experience that you can ever have."

JANET RENO

HOW TO MASSAGE YOUR CHILD'S EXTENSOR MUSCLES

APPROXIMATE MASSAGE TIME: 8-10 MINUTES

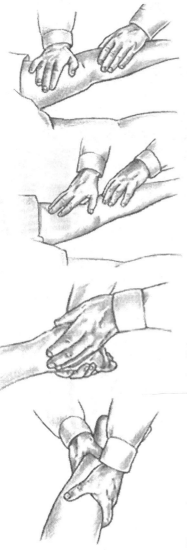

1 Have your child lay on his stomach and position yourself at the bottom of his feet. Put some oil on your hands and rub them together. Spread the oil all the way up the back of his right leg—cover the foot, calf, behind the knee, and up the thigh, using medium pressure.

2 When the leg is thoroughly oiled, use your fingertips to lightly rake down the entire leg, one hand following the other. Repeat this stroke several times to cover the entire back of the leg.

3 Now take his right foot in your right hand. In a squeezing motion, spread the skin and muscles on the outside of the foot, moving toward the inside of the foot. Stimulate the soft skin by raking your fingertips across the sole. Alternate the stimulation by using your knuckles for some of the strokes.

4 Now wrap both of your hands around his right leg just above the ankle, making sure your palms are against the front part of the leg. Using a slow rope-climbing motion—hand over hand—massage up and then down his leg. As you complete this stroke, be sure to use firm pressure to extend the skin and muscles of the leg.

5 Repeat steps 1 through 4 on her left leg.

6 Apply more oil to your hands and warm it. Return your attention to his right leg. Place both of your thumbs together in the center of the back of his leg, right above the ankle. Using a strong kneading motion with your thumbs, spread the oil out to each side. Do this all the way up the entire leg until you reach the buttocks, working always from the center outward.

7 Oil your hands and repeat step 6 on the right leg.

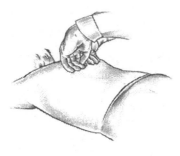

8 Now stand on one side of your child's body, with your child still on his stomach. Using your right hand (palm and fingertips), and starting on the left side of his lower back, spread oil up to the shoulders, across the spine, and back down the right side. Then, reverse your direction, moving from the right side up, across the spine, and down the left. Repeat this exercise two or three times.

9 Place your hands at the small of his back, right in the middle. Stroke the fingers of both hands in zigzag motion up and down either side of the spine. Let the skin slide between your fingers as you go. Do this a few times. When you reach the top of the shoulders, spread your fingers out to the sides and across the shoulder blades. Bring your hands together in the center of the spine and follow the spine back down to the middle of the lower back with your fingertips. After you've done this a few times, lightly brush your fingertips down past his back and over her legs, driving all the tension out of his toes.

10 Ask your child to turn over so that he is now lying on his back with his knees up and his feet flat. Have him raise his pelvis up and position your right hand, palm up, on his tailbone (just above the buttocks). Lay your left hand on the front of his torso, just below the rib cage. Now with your right hand, begin to lightly stretch the muscles of his lower back by gently pulling down on the area two to three inches above the tail bone, applying slight pressure with your left hand from the top. Then gently lower his pelvis.

11 Lastly, massage the back of your child's neck.

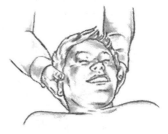

While he's still on his back, stand behind him with his head facing you. Cradle the back of his neck with both of your hands. Gently move your hands up and down either side of his neck, lightly pulling on the muscles as you move, lengthening the spine.

TIPS FOR PARENTS

1. HOW FAR CAN YOU GO?

Take your child out for a run. Every day for a week run the same distance. The next week tell your child you are going to go farther and set a new landmark to run to. Then, the next week, go even farther. This will be a stretch for your child, but one that is possible to attain. He will be developing physical strength while also learning how to create and attain new goals.

2. FASTER/SLOWER

This can also be applied to almost everything your child will do. For example, when he is learning to count, tell him to count from one to ten aloud as fast as he can. Then have him count from one to ten as slow as he can. Tell him to pay attention to his body while counting. Next, have him count backward from ten to one, as fast as he can and as slow as he can. You can add many variations to this game.

3. WIN/LOSE

It is important for your child to learn how to deal with winning as well as losing. This game is quite simple. Separate a bunch of marbles into two piles on the floor, designating a pile for each of you. The person who picks up her marbles the fastest wins. Before you begin, however, let your child pick whether he wants to win or lose. Whoever chooses to win, the other has to let win. Your child, being no dummy, will always choose to win. So you should encourage him to let you win every once in a while. (This will come in very handy further on down the road in that argument on who gets the car!)

HEAD AND NECK
A NEW PERSPECTIVE

Perspective is a funny animal. For better or worse, it shapes our lives. And as it is through the lens of our unique perspective that we view the world, each of us has some measure of control over our own reality.

Your perspective on the world derives from your physical and mental behavior. Someone who stands upright and thinks positive thoughts will develop a healthier perspective than someone who slouches down and complains constantly. Also, a positive perspective will allow flexibility and growth—both physically and emotionally.

So it makes sense to say that by expanding the scope of your perspective, you can enlarge your world. When you do expand your perspective, life becomes full of opportunities. Of course, the reverse is also true: if you do not try to see past the self-imposed blinders of a narrow perspective, life can become stagnant.

But expanding your perspective—like most worthwhile things in life—is easier said than done.

An important axiom to remember is this: You never know what you can do until you try. We risk never realizing our full potential as long as we remain in the shadow cast by narrow thought habits and conditioning. But by challenging your perspective once in a while—by having the confidence to try something new—you will actually increase the scope of your perspective, and therefore the world around you.

Unfortunately, many people are unaware that they possess this power to transform their perspective on the world. But it is a fact that human beings—both as individuals and as a species—can change their perspective for the better. For example, over tens of thousands of years the human body has evolved toward a more upright position. This change of physical perspective led to positive changes in mental capabilities. The same can be said for individuals today: by improving your physical perspective, you will enhance your mental capabilities.

Massage will offer a new perspective for you and your family. And it will also open up a whole new world of possibilities, many of which are not yet even imagined. Currently, the idea of massage for children is not a popular developmental tool. But once you make it a major part of your life, your perspective of the world—and your child's perspective—will expand dramatically.

HOW TO MASSAGE YOUR BABY'S HEAD AND NECK

APPROXIMATE MASSAGE TIME: 4 MINUTES

It is well known that babies' heads are fragile—especially around the "soft spot"—yet this does not mean that you should not touch this area. Simply use your best judgment and proceed with care.

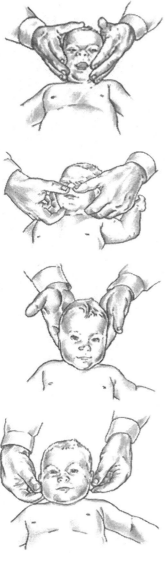

1 Lay your baby down on her back and stand at the top of her head. Lightly oil your hands, rubbing them together to warm the oil. Before beginning the massage, spread oil on your baby's face, being careful to avoid the eyes. Use the pads of your thumb and forefingers to gently spread the oil, always working from the center of the face out. Make sure you cover the entire forehead, nose, upper lip, cheeks, and chin.

2 Start by using your forefingers to massage and stretch the area around her mouth. Begin with your thumbs together in the center, just below the nose, and move them outward and around the lips. Now perform this center-to-sides motion with your thumbs on his chin. Move slowly and explore the contours of your child's face, always remembering to keep your touch gentle and light. Direct the stroke from the center of the chin along the jawline and ending at the ears.

3 Reach under your baby's head and place the first two fingers of both hands at the base of her neck, centered on the spine. Slowly spread your fingers out to the sides and up to the ears. Do this three or four times, always working from the center outward.

4 Now use your thumb and forefingers to gently massage the earlobes. Lightly pinch and pull the lobe between your thumb and forefingers to relieve tension. This will feel great to your baby. The earlobe is part of the hearing mechanism—loud noises or sudden noises startle your baby, causing this area to tense up, inhibiting or limiting hearing.

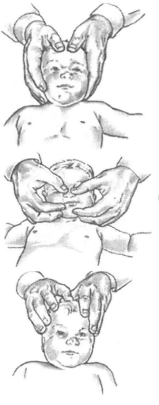

5 Place your thumb tips together at her hairline (or where the hairline will be once some hair grows in!). Slowly and gently sweep your thumbs off to the side of the head, gradually moving down to the tops of the eyebrows.

6 Place your thumbs on the bridge of the nose. Sweep the thumbs down either side of the nose and across the cheeks. Repeat several times.

7 End the massage by gently massaging the scalp with your fingertips. Lightly caress your baby's head, moving your fingertips around the top and sides. Place your fingertips lightly on his eyebrows and gently brush the temples with your thumbs.

TIPS FOR PARENTS

1. CHANGE THE MOBILE IN YOUR BABY'S CRIB

Any baby who looks at the same old mobile, with the same objects, day after day, may eventually become bored. Consider changing the objects that hang from it and your baby will stay interested. You can do this every so often to help energize her brain and transform the familiar into something new.

2. TEACH YOUR BABY SHAPES

Cut out different shapes and paste them on large pieces of drawing paper or sheets of cardboard. Use one shape for each sheet. Show her one sheet at a time for a few seconds saying the corresponding name of each shape. Be sure to use your imagination and make it fun.

3. TEACH YOUR BABY COLORS

One way to do this is to go to a paint store and collect different paint swatches. You can then group the swatches by color and mount them on large sheets of cardboard. This way you can introduce your baby to a whole spectrum of shades! Of course, you should start off slowly. Let your baby become familiar with basic colors—red, orange, yellow, green, blue, purple, brown, and black.

HOW TO MASSAGE YOUR CHILD'S HEAD AND NECK

APPROXIMATE MASSAGE TIME: 4 MINUTES

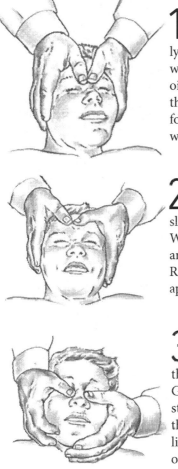

1 Have your child lie on his back and position yourself at the top of his head. Lightly oil your hands, rubbing them together to warm the oil. Begin to spread a light layer of oil over his entire face, using caution around the eye area. Use the pads of your thumb and forefingers to gently spread the oil, always working from the center of the face out.

2 Place your thumbs together in the middle of his forehead. Then slowly separate them, sliding them across either side of his forehead. With light strokes work toward his temples, and massage that area with a circular motion. Repeat this sequence using your fingers, and apply a slightly harder touch.

3 Next, repeat the above motions on his cheeks, first with the thumbs and then the fingers, starting at either side of his nose. Gently use your forefingers to massage and stretch the area around his mouth—start at the lips and rub your fingers away from the lips. Place your thumbs together in the center of the upper lip just below the nose, and move them outward and around the area outside of the lips.

4 Now repeat this motion with your thumbs on his chin, starting at the center with both thumbs and spreading them out along the jawline. Try using different amounts of pressure with each stroke—your child will enjoy the variety of stimulation.

5 To massage your child's neck, place the first two fingers of both hands under the base of his skull, in the middle of the spine. Slowly spread your fingers out to the sides and up to the ears. Do this a few times, always working from the center outward.

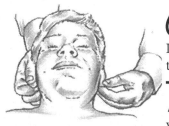

6 Now you can use your thumb and forefingers to gently massage the earlobes. Lightly pinch and pull the lobes between your thumbs and forefingers to relieve tension.

7 End the massage by gently massaging his scalp with your fingers, lightly caressing your child's entire head in a swirling, circular motion.

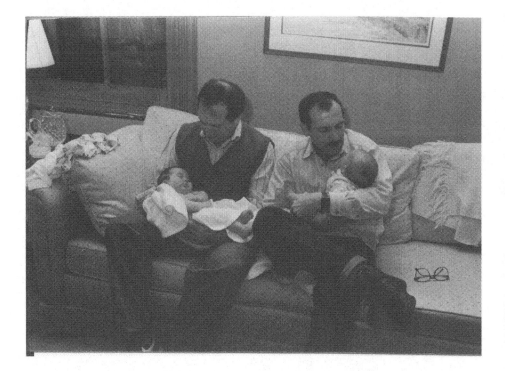

TIPS FOR PARENTS

1. A TIME TO LEARN

Children love to learn about animals, dinosaurs, art, flowers, flags of the world—just about anything you can think of. You can educate your little one about any one of these thing by presenting them with little bits of information. Find posters or pictures in any store, art book, or magazine. Cut them out and paste them onto sheets of paper. Then show your toddler three to five different pictures, explaining each in simple terms, from three to five categories a day. Every day be sure to add new objects of interest. Talk to him about what he's looking at. You'll be raising a child with a lively interest in the world around him and with a vocabulary beyond that of the average child of his age. This exercise takes just minutes to prepare for and a few more minutes to fulfill. But it will provide infinite results as your child will truly enjoy learning—now, and for the rest of his life.

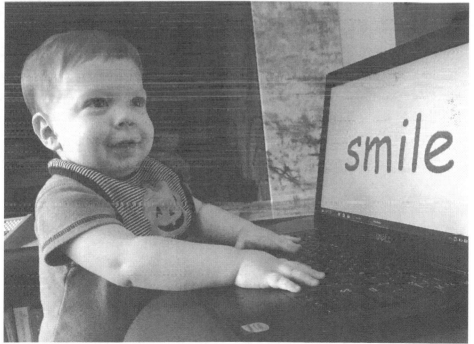

Zelek enjoying www.brillkids.com, www.brillbaby.com.

LOWER BODY

BALANCE AND LIVING IN THE PRESENT

Balance in our bodies is closely related to the balance in our lives. A balanced body—one that receives a good diet, regular exercise, and healthy human touch—will promote a more balanced life in general. When the cares of the body are met, one can pursue all kinds of interests with vim and vigor. Conversely, if the cares of the body are not met, then the life in general suffers.

Think of balance as a resting state from which you respond to the world around you. Naturally, every response to stimuli causes a temporary imbalance, but the body quickly returns to a balanced state when the encounter has been met successfully. However, if your response does not produce a successful outcome, you will undoubtedly experience stress. Furthermore, when unsuccessful encounters start to pile up, your body and life may take on a pattern of imbalance. This imbalance can be seen in your posture and your actions.

Now this is not to say that you must never experience failure in order to avoid becoming unbalanced. A "successful encounter" means that you have reacted to something as best you could. Life is full of ups and downs—your healthy reaction to both ups and downs will help you maintain balance in your life.

Our lives, in fact, reflect a constant struggle to maintain balance—balance between work and family, balancing our finances, balancing our private and public lives, and so on.

Every incomplete or inadequate encounter ends up being internalized, and together these bad experiences develop into general restrictions that cause imbalance—both physically and emotionally. These restrictions turn into "knots" in our lives and "knots" in our bodies. They are what we commonly call "baggage." The more baggage you carry, the more weighted down you become. You know how much baggage you have by seeing how much of your life is influenced by events of the past or apprehension about the future.

But you can avoid and eliminate baggage! The best way to rid yourself of excess baggage is to live in the present—unencumbered by past failures or future fears. Live one day at a time! The very powerful contact that is massage can help focus you and your children into the present, pushing that baggage deep into the subconscious.

Moreover, you can communicate with your child about his baggage, thus enabling him to let go of it. The combination of physical massage and intimate communication provides a powerful way to let go—and to return to a state of balance.

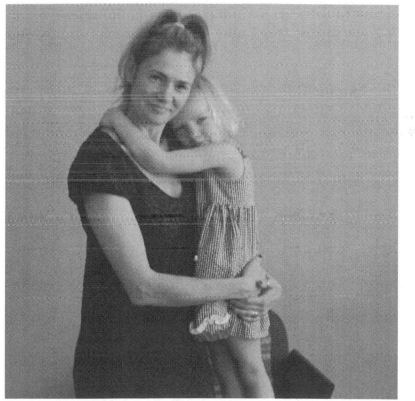

Stephanie and Heidie after Rolfing sessions.

HOW TO MASSAGE YOUR BABY'S LOWER BODY

APPROXIMATE MASSAGE TIME: 6 MINUTES

Lay your baby on her back and position yourself at her feet. Put some oil on your hands and rub them together to warm the oil. Lightly cover the entire lower body with oil, including the pelvis, thighs, knees, lower legs, and feet.

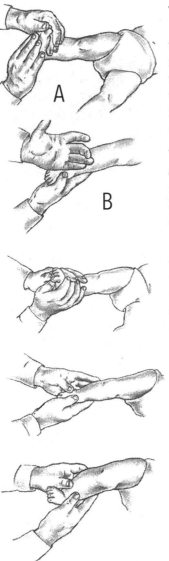

A

B

1 Begin the massage at her feet (illustration A). Slide your fingertips up the bottom of the foot from the heel, and then to each toe, remembering to wiggle your fingers in between the toes. Use the outside of your hand to rub the outside of the foot (illustration B) and the inside of your hand on the inside of the foot (the instep). Repeat on the other foot.

2 Place your thumbs on the sole of the foot at the tip of the toes and, beginning at the midline, work toward the outside with one hand and the inside with the other. Progress down toward the heel with each stroke.

3 Now use your thumbs to work on the top of the foot. Use only enough pressure to feel the muscles and tissue stretching a little under your fingers. Start at the midline at the tips of the toes and work toward the outside of the foot with one hand and the inside with the other, flicking your thumb tips off the foot at its sides. Repeat this motion as you move up the foot to the ankle.

Then repeat the entire process two or three times. Then repeat the process on the other foot.

4 Now move up the leg. Continue using your thumbs and, starting at the top of the ankle, kneed the muscles as though you were spreading modeling clay over your baby's ankle. Spread the muscles around the ankle, down and to the outside with one hand and toward the inside with the other. Repeat on the other ankle.

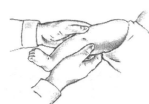

5 Return to the top of the ankle. Place both thumb tips on the shinbone and spread them down either side of the calf muscle, repeating the motion as you gradually move up to the knee area. Once you get to the knee, return directly to the ankle and repeat this step two or three times. After the second or third repetition, take a few minutes to explore the knee with your fingertips—wiggle the knee around a bit, but very gently. Then administer this step on the other leg.

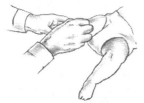

6 Now move up the thigh in the same manner that you moved up the shin, always starting with the thumbs at the midline of the thigh. Repeat a few times and then switch legs.

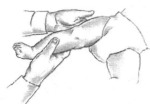

7 Reach around to the back of the leg with one hand while stabilizing the leg with your other hand on the pelvis. With your free hand, gently glide your palm all the way down to the heel in one swift motion from the upper thigh to the ankle, flicking your hand off her heel at the end as if to flick tension away. Repeat on the other leg.

8 Returning to the heel, stabilize the leg with one hand on the foot and glide your free hand in one sweeping motion up the back of the leg to the pelvis area. Then smooth your palm over the pelvis and back around to the lower back and buttocks, and then quickly sweep the hand back down to the ankle. Repeat this procedure on the other leg. Even though you are not ready for a full body massage, you want your baby to have the feeling that the upper and lower parts of her body are one unit. This connection will be made by sweeping over the pelvis, around to the buttocks, and down to the ankle in one swift motion.

TIPS FOR PARENTS

1. BALANCE THE BABY

It's never too early for your baby to learn about balance. Teach her about the symmetrical aspects of her body—right and left and top and bottom. Have fun with this. You may even make up a little song or rhyme. Remember, the more your baby or child knows about her body, the more in balance she will be in relation to her surroundings.

2. NO TIME LIKE THE PRESENT

A great way to live in the present is to be aware of your body. Feel your energy. Wiggle your toes. Encourage your baby to do the same. Touch her toes and ask her how it feels. She will be responding to your touch specifically, not just to the typical question of "How are you?" This way, she will understand that "How are you?" can be answered based on the present moment, not just as a reflex.

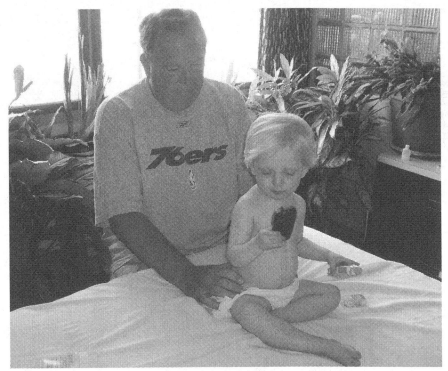

Rolfing Cloe one more time.

HOW TO MASSAGE YOUR CHILD'S LOWER BODY
APPROXIMATE MASSAGE TIME: 6 MINUTES

Have your child lie on his back and position yourself at the bottom of his feet. Put some oil on your hands and rub them together to warm the oil. Gently apply a light layer of oil over the feet, legs, and pelvic area of both legs. Use more oil whenever necessary.

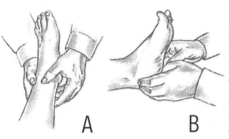

A B

1 Start off by massaging his foot (illustration A). Briefly kneed each part—around the ankles, the heel, the sole, and up to the toes—with your fingertips and thumbs. Then place your thumb tips at the center point of the heel (illustration B) and lightly knead the sole of the foot from the center outward, using both thumbs on either side. Work your way up to the tips of the toes with each successive stroke. Repeat on the other foot.

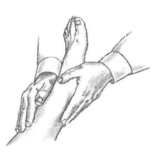

2 Place your fingertips and thumb tips together just above the ankle on the center of the shinbone of one leg. Using your fingertips to apply solid pressure, work the skin and muscles of the calf down to either side; let your fingertips slide right off the leg in a flicking action at the end of the stroke. Your thumb tips should remain planted on the shinbone. Repeat this stroke as you move up the leg to the knee. Take a minute to explore the knee with your fingertips, then repeat the entire process on the other leg.

3 Now place your fingertips together at the top of the knee. Move up across the thigh in the same manner that you moved up over the calf and shin—always starting each dual stroke at the midline of the thigh—and end the strokes at the pelvis. You can apply more pressure to these strokes since there is more muscle to work over.

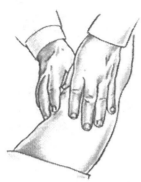

4 Once you reach the top of the thigh, brush the palm of one hand over the pelvis and around to the back of the leg, then gently but swiftly glide that hand across the back of the leg and all the way down to the heel, flicking your fingertips off the heel at the end of the stroke. Repeat steps 3 and 4 two or three times, and then duplicate the process on the other leg.

5 Return to the top of the ankle and explore it momentarily on either side with your fingertips. Now, using your palms, swiftly glide one hand followed by the other up across the front of his leg, over the pelvis, and around to the lower back. Massage his lower back with the fingertips of one hand for a minute or two—this will create a conscious connection between his upper and lower body—and then finally sweep the palm of one hand down the back of the leg and off the heel. Repeat this final step on the other leg.

TIPS FOR PARENTS

1. BOTH SIDES ARE "RIGHT"

Help your child develop ambidextrous qualities. Most of us have a dominant side. We label ourselves as "right-handed" or "left-handed." We can usually throw a ball better, kick harder, and write clearer, with one side of the body as compared to the other. We all have the capacity, however, to develop equal capabilities (or close to equal) with both our right and left sides.

Encourage your child to use both of his limbs equally. This will help him become more balanced and gain greater control over her body. Have him write his name with his right hand. Then have him do it with his left. This may at first be a challenge to your child, making him frustrated. So try to infuse fun into the activity by playing along with him. Write your name with your right hand, then again with your left. Let your child see the differences between the two. He is sure to giggle when she sees what Mommy's or Daddy's "opposite hand" handwriting looks like.

This "right/left" game can be applied to almost anything—tying shoelaces, brushing teeth, or combing hair, for instance. And the more he works with each hand equally, the easier it will become!

2. ACTION/REACTION

You know the theory that for every action there is an equal and opposite reaction. What better time to teach your child this than when he's a toddler. Your child has no doubt learned this to some extent. For instance, if he leaves his toys all over the floor, Mom will not be a happy camper. But if he picks up after herself, as he has been told, Mom is appreciative. Help him understand how this law of cause and effect applies to all other areas of life.

UPPER BODY
SELF-ESTEEM

A recent study on self-esteem (funded by the State Assembly in California) found that the more someone contributed to the needs of other people, the better they felt. The study also demonstrated that one of the most frustrating circumstances in people's lives is the feeling that the future is shaping them instead of them shaping the future. These two points are related because they reveal that a person can positively affect their own well-being and self-esteem by becoming proactive in their life.

The question for you is: How are you going to raise your child to grow up feeling good about herself?

In today's climate of rapid changes and puzzling challenges, it is important for your child to know when and how to respond to a variety of situations.

A number of years ago in California, I met John Vasconcellos, the state assemblyman who founded the funding in California for the study of self-esteem. The study ultimately determined that everyone, no matter their circumstances, has something to contribute and that when you reach out to make a difference, you feel better about yourself.

I have been doing this most of my adult life. Serving those in need has proven to be a great comfort to me during my own difficult trials in life, and I've been privileged to see the fruits of that service expand in ways I couldn't imagine at the time. (You can read more about this in the "Team Children" and "My Story" sections at the end of the book.)

Children—along with many adults—can be their own worst critics. Children don't need their parents contributing to their sense of insecurity or alienation. What they do need is lots and lots of positive input and a firm establishment of moral standards.

Have you ever met someone who was overloved or overacknowledged? Not likely! We all like a pat on the back when we've done a good job or when we've tried our best. Reaching out and touching your child is a significant way to send that message. You'll see it paying off later in life when they reach out to their friends and when their friends return the feelings of warmth and companionship. The ability to reach out like this comes part and parcel with having strong self-esteem.

So when you think of the phrase, "reach out and touch someone," try to remember that it doesn't have to be limited to making a phone call. Actually do it!

"Children are not casual guests in our home. They have been loaned to us temporarily for the purpose of loving them and instilling a foundation of values on which their future lives will be built."

JAMES DOBSON

HOW TO MASSAGE YOUR BABY'S UPPER BODY
APPROXIMATE MASSAGE TIME: 12–15 MINUTES

Put some oil on your hands and rub them together to warm your hands and the oil. Tell your baby that you are now going to massage her hands, arms, and shoulders. Place your baby on her back and position yourself on her right side.

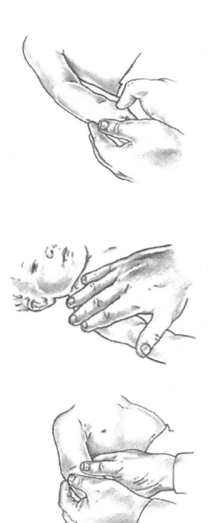

1 Begin by using both of your hands to spread the oil on both sides of your baby's left hand. Make sure that you put oil on and between each finger. Using just your fingertips, begin to rub circles on the back of her hand. Then gently rub circles on her palm. Explore each crease, each finger joint, and each tiny fingertip with your own fingertips. Make sure you distinguish and explore the front, back, and sides of each finger, but spend only about five seconds on each finger. As you finish with each finger, brush the tension out by flicking your fingertips off the end of her fingertips.

2 Next, holding her left hand in your left hand, with your right hand begin to spread oil up the right arm all the way to the shoulder. Let your hand glide up the wrist, the forearm, the crook of the elbow, and the upper arm. When you reach the shoulder, place your palm on the underside of the arm and gently slide your hand down all the way to the palm.

3 You want her to start distinguishing the differences between her fingers, wrist, elbow, and shoulder. So with just your fingertips, slowly work your way up the arm again, lingering at each joint and mentioning the name of the joint as you trace the curves lightly with your fingertips. Then work back down to her hand and in a sweeping motion brush all the tension out of the hand and fingers. Repeat steps 1 through 3 on the other arm.

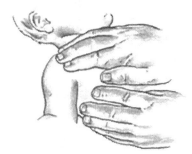

4 Put some more oil on your hands and rub them together to warm it. Spread the oil on the chest and sides, starting at the neck and ending at the abdomen. Stimulate this area by rubbing lightly from the midpoint out to the sides and off the body, again moving from the neck down.

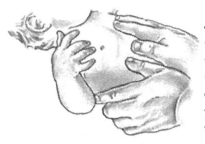

5 Place both hands on your baby's chest on either side of the sternum, and gently slide your fingertips up the chest, over the shoulders, and down the arms all the way to the hands in one sweeping motion. Gently let your baby's hands slip out of your hands. You may also choose to give the hands a little squeeze as a sign of love and encouragement.

6 The next step is to turn your baby around so that you are standing at her head. Pour a small amount of oil onto your palms and rub them together. Using your thumb tips and fingertips, start at the center of the forehead and spread the oil on the forehead ever so slightly. Gently place your fingertips on the center of her forehead and rub little circles from the center out to the temples.

7 Place both hands under your baby's head and just let it relax there. Use your thumbs to softly massage the temples. Then, gently pull your hands out away from her body, feeling the neck stretching ever so slightly, and lay her head gently back down.

TIPS FOR PARENTS

1. MAKE YOUR BABY STRONG

Lay your baby on her back. Hold her feet in your hands and pull her legs up into the air. Now push her legs down toward her body and encourage her to resist by pushing her legs toward you (she will likely do this as a natural reaction anyway). As she pushes back, tell her how strong her legs are!

2. SAY THANK YOU!

Realize that your baby contributes as much to your well-being as you do to hers. Parents often are so caught up in providing for their baby that they fail to realize how much support their baby is actually giving them. And yet, the child's emotional needs include giving to her parents as much as they will let her. When you sense that your baby wants to give back to you, be as open and receptive as you possibly can. And say, "Thank you!"

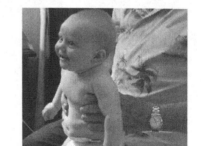

MADISON BEFORE ROLFING

MEET THE BABIES

MADISON AFTER 4 ROLFING SESSIONS

HOW TO MASSAGE YOUR CHILD'S UPPER BODY
APPROXIMATE MASSAGE TIME: 12–15 MINUTES

Put some oil on your hands and rub them together to warm the oil. Tell your child that you are now going to massage his hands, arms, chest, and shoulders—areas that are intimately related to strength, confidence, and self-esteem.

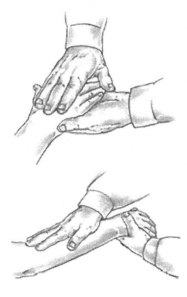

1 Have your child lie on his back, and stand by his right side. Spread the oil on the top of his right hand while spreading oil on her palm with your other hand. Make sure that you put oil on and between each finger. Using just your fingertips, begin to rub circles first on the top of his hand, and then on his palm. As you massage the top of the hand, use your fingertips to slowly brush all the tension out of the hand and fingers.

2 Holding his right hand in your left hand for support, use your right hand to spread oil up the top of the arm all the way to the shoulder. Then work back down on the underside of the arm by gently sliding your hand all the way down to the palm, moving your left hand out of the way as you go.

3 Using just the fingertips of both hands, begin to distinguish the hand from the wrist and the wrist from the elbow. Gently use your fingertips to trace the contour of the wrist. Then place his hand in your left hand, and with just the slightest amount of pressure walk the fingers of your right hand up to the elbow. Trace the contours of the elbow. Then use your fingertips to sweep all the tension down the arm and out of the hand, flicking your fingertips off the end of his fingertips.

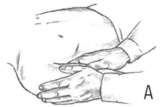

A

B

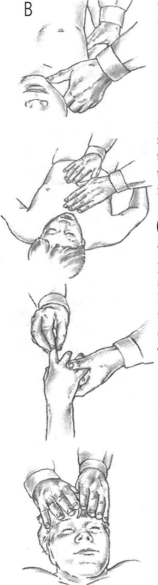

4 Warm more oil in your hands and spread it over the upper arm (illustration A). Walk your fingertips from the elbow up the arm to the shoulder. When you get to the top of the shoulder, slide your fingers over the shoulder and across the side of the neck (illustration B), and then back to the outer part of the shoulder. Then swiftly sweep your fingertips down the arm to the hands and let all that tension flow right out the tips of his fingers. Repeat this step two or three times.

5 Next, put a little oil on the chest and sides. Use long, straight strokes to stimulate the skin and muscles up along the chest and sides, starting from the waist and ending at the shoulder blade. Make two or three strokes, using your fingertips to apply firm, even pressure.

6 Grasp his hand in yours and begin to distinguish each finger and each part of the finger. Use only your fingertips. Make sure you distinguish and explore the front, back, and sides of each finger, but spend only five seconds on each finger. When you have completely massaged the hand, quickly stroke your entire palm back up the entire arm to the shoulder, and then glide it back down again.

7 The final step in this important massage routine is to massage the forehead. Using your fingertips, spread some oil on his forehead ever so slightly. Then gently place your fingertips just below the hairline and rub little circles from the center of the forehead to the outside. Gradually move the strokes down toward the eyebrows.

8 Next place both hands under your child's head and let it rest there. You can use your thumbs to gently massage the temples. Then, gently pull your hands out as you feel the skin and muscles of the neck stretching ever so slightly. Slowly remove your hands and lay his head back down to complete the massage.

TIPS FOR PARENTS

1. BRACHIATION LADDER

A brachiation ladder is one with multiple horizontal rungs where the child is able to move from one rung to the next using his or her hands only.

The body is suspended and elongated, thus stretching out the spine and entire body in the process. This exercise also complements any strength-training program you may initiate. It also has a number of developmental benefits. Research has found that while swinging from one rung to the next, the brain works left, then right, in a perfect alternating pattern, which, neurologically, is an important part of growing up. You can learn more about brachiation ladders and where to purchase them at the Institute for the Achievement of Human Potential: www.iahp.org

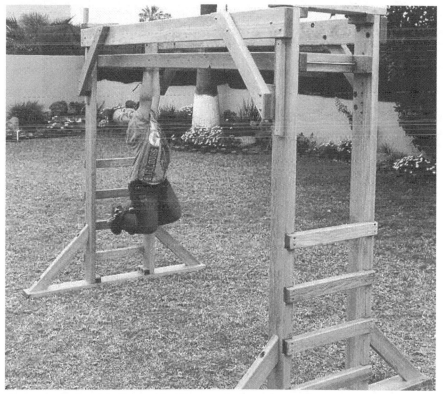

Photo credit: Raul F. Hernandez Forever Redwood www.foreverredwood.com

2. CREATE A NEW CHALLENGE

From time to time, about every three to four months, create a new challenge for your child which will cause him to go beyond where he is now in his motor development. For instance, if you're playing catch with a big ball, find a smaller ball. If he is capable of putting together a six-piece puzzle, give him a ten-piece puzzle. If your child thinks he can't do something, work with him until he can.

This can sometimes be a painstaking process, but in the end the child will realize that you only lose if you quit. What a valuable lesson for him to learn at such an early age!

3. DON'T DISCOURAGE CRYING

As your child begins to grow and take on more challenges, there will be more opportunity to hurt himself or get hurt. The old belief that only sissies cry is actually harmful. Children should be encouraged to show their emotions. Here's a suggestion: When your child gets hurt, encourage him to cry no matter what his age. Explain to him that it is really good to let go of his feelings instead of keeping them locked inside. Most importantly, comfort his in her pain. Moreover, when he takes on a challenge that is beyond his capabilities, let him know that it's okay to fail. The most important thing is that he tried his best.

4. ACKNOWLEDGE WHAT YOUR CHILD CAN DO

Children are often called "rug rats" because they generally crawl on the floor, yet they always get in your hair! Children love to participate in making a difference, making a mess, and being involved. If you constantly tell your child, "Don't do this" and "Don't do that," he will never grow up with a sense of what he can do or be. So, accentuate the positive. Encourage your child to do all he is capable of in terms of physical and mental activities. If he gets in your hair, be grateful that he is an active, healthy child.

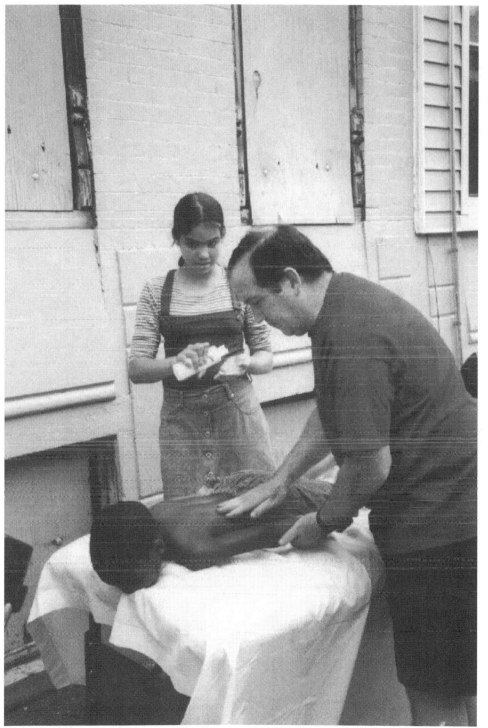
Teaching low-income kids the value of Rolfing/massage.

CONNECTING THE WHOLE BODY
COMPLETION

Completion means to make whole, to bring together, to heal. Completion can be thought of as an attitude or a posture—it is a state of being that you must continuously strive to achieve. The more complete you are, the more whole you can be, and therefore, the more healthy. Counteracting this sense of completion are the attitudes and tensions we have mentioned throughout this book—the things that we hold in or have held back. Massage is one of the best tools you can use to avoid holding things back, or to release the things you're holding in.

Up until now, we have covered massage from the point of view of separate, isolated body areas. Now we want to approach the body as a whole, with every part being connected. Also, it is important to remember that our life experiences are as much a part of our body as our arms and legs are. Whenever you get something off your chest, you let it go and become free of its hold. Whenever you take a stand, you become firmer on your feet. And when you hold your head up straighter, you will expand your perspective.

As we've discussed, in order to solve a problem you need to be conscious of the perspective from which you are viewing the problem. In fact, your whole family can benefit from learning to hone their perspective.

One way to achieve this is to hold a regular "completion" meeting with your family members in which you talk about everything that was positive during the preceding week, as well as everything that could have been improved upon. Through this meeting, all family members will get their triumphs and frustrations—however minor—out in the open. This will help every member of your family understand their own lives and each other's lives, and to get a clearer sense of the "big picture." After all, as the great philosopher Plato said, "The life which is unexamined is not worth living."

As your family participation and communication increases and solidifies, you'll be pleasantly surprised by the happy, healthy atmosphere that will be created. Your friends will wonder at the sense of well-being that you radiate.

Moreover, when you start to give your child this final, full body massage, you should be considering the ideas imparted in the previous chapters. Synthesize those ideas to reveal the importance of maintaining your child's sense of wholeness and completion.

HOW TO GIVE YOUR BABY OR CHILD A FULL-BODY MASSAGE

APPROXIMATE MASSAGE TIME: 15 MINUTES

Put oil on your hands and rub them together to warm the oil. To begin, place both your hands on your child's chest. Use your palms to spread the oil up to his shoulders and around her neck. Then cover his arms, hands, and fingers.

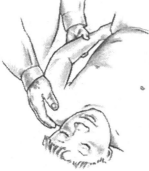

1 Take his lower left arm in your hand for support. Cup your hand around his arm just under the shoulder, and quickly glide your hand down his arm to the wrist. Remove your support hand and complete the stroke over his hands and fingers, letting all accumulated tension flow out of his body. You should apply gentle pressure to the skin as you move down the arm. Repeat this stroke two or three times.

2 Pull each joint of the arm (illustration A). Hold the upper arm for support and grasp the lower arm to pull out the elbow joint. Hold the lower arm and grasp the hand (illustration B) to pull out the wrist joint. Hold the hand and then grasp each fingertip (one at a time) to pull out the finger joints. Then repeat steps 1 and 2 on the other arm.

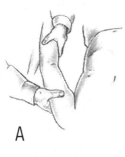

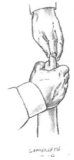

A   B

3 Spread oil across the front, sides, and back of his leg all the way down to and including his entire foot. Raise his leg in the air and use your free palm to sweep down the back of his leg down to his heel, across the foot, and sweep all the tension out the toes. Lower his leg and sweep your palm down the front of his leg from the top of the thigh to the tip of the toes. Repeat these motions on her other leg.

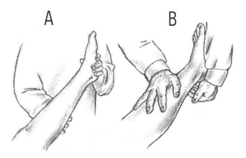

A   B

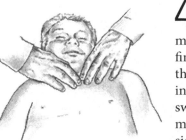

4 Apply more oil to your hands and warm it. Now, starting just below the chin, massage your child's neck with your forefingers using short sweeping motions from the center out to the sides. Continue brushing the tension out of his body with short sweeping motions along his ribcage as you move down to his waist. You can cover both sides at the same time using both of your hands.

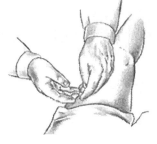

5 Continue the short sweeping motions down his legs, each stroke moving from the center point of the leg off to the sides. Concentrate on one leg at a time, using both of your hands on either side of the leg. Finish these strokes at the tips of the toes, then repeat on the other leg.

6 Now, turn him over on his stomach. Warm more oil in your hands and apply it evenly to his shoulders, back, and legs. With your fingertips resting on his shoulder blades, drag your hands down his back in a serpentine motion. Start with both hands at the spine and with each new stroke move farther out toward the sides. Continue the serpentine motion down the back of his legs to his toes. (You can do both legs at the same time, one with either hand.)

7 Return your fingertips to his shoulder blades. Use short sweeping motions from the center of the back out to the sides to brush the tension out of the body. Spread your fingers out and stretch the various segments of the back area with firm pressure as you move down.

8 Now turn your baby over on his back. Warm more oil in your hands. Using your thumbs, start in the middle of his forehead and sweep down along the hairline to her ears. Take his ears between your thumb and forefinger and massage them. With your thumbs and/or fingertips, massage his cheeks, nose, upper lip, and down to her chin. The strokes on his face can be accomplished with just a fingertip or two. You should adjust the amount of pressure you apply to the face according to your child's needs.

9 Now reach underneath his with one hand and rest it on the small of his back. With your other hand on her abdomen, begin to pull her spine down to lengthen it. Congratulate his and tell him he has just had a full body massage and that he has a complete, perfect body.

TIPS FOR YOUR BABY AND CHILD
WHAT "TO DO"

Make a "things to do" list at the beginning of every day. At the end of every day, check off what you have accomplished and what still has to be done. Encourage each family member to make a list each day—this should become a very important habit. Otherwise, you'll all carry everything you have to do around in your heads—a perfect scenario for forgetting!

> "When inquiry is suppressed by previous knowledge, or by the authority and experience of another, then learning becomes mere imitation, and imitation causes a human being to repeat what is learned without experiencing it."
>
> –J. KRISHNAMURTI

PART THREE
SPECIAL CONCERNS

WHILE MASSAGE IS USEFUL AND BENEFICIAL to a "normal" child, regular massage is crucial to the child with special concerns. Touch is one of the most ignored, but critical, elements for such children. Along with allowing deep relaxation, which is always beneficial, massage can help meet the specific needs of babies born prematurely or with some other birth trauma, as well as children with illness or disabilities. Some of the benefits of massage for these children include:

• Providing a comfortable and enjoyable experience. This is especially important if your child is receiving uncomfortable or painful medical treatment.

• Strengthening and facilitating a "normal" parent and child connection. It is natural for parents of a "special needs" child to experience a variety of emotions, including confusion, denial, guilt, anger, wishful thinking, depression, intellectualization, and acceptance. This can inadvertently influence interactions with their child. Massage is an expression of pure love and acceptance.

• Stimulating the immune system and the circulatory system.

• Aiding the digestive process and relieving constipation.

• Increasing trust and acceptance of touch ("Special needs" children tend to be socially isolated and are touched less than "normal" children. It is important for them to be able to both give and receive tactile stimulation.)

• Encouraging deep breathing and deep relaxation.

• Normalizing muscle tone and preventing contracture.

• Increasing body awareness and body acceptance.

• Increasing mobility and flexibility.

• Relieving muscle fatigue and strain.

You can begin massaging your child immediately after birth, following the techniques offered in this book. Be sure to use common sense, talk to your child, and watch for signs of discomfort. Of course, you'll want to consult your physician about any extra precautions you should take. For premature babies, massage offers enormous benefits.

Unfortunately, this fact has not been widely accepted by the medical community. One exception is the Touch Research Institute in Miami—backed by a tremendous amount of funding from the pharmaceutical firm Johnson & Johnson™—which has begun to scientifically document the impact massage can have on premature babies. Their studies have found that premature babies massaged briefly three times a day for ten days gain 47% more weight than equally ill infants. Moreover, they leave the hospital an average of six days earlier. Massage stabilizes the babies' heart rate and breathing, and most importantly, it helps them fall into a deep sleep, which is fundamental to weight gain. Although this research has been widely reported in various publications, it seems to be making little or no difference in most neonatal intensive care units.

It's up to you, the parent (and that applies to both mother and father) to make sure the baby gets the touching she needs and deserves right after birthing. No one will love, care, or be as committed to your baby as you will. Do not expect that the traditional obstetrician to stress, or even mention, the importance of touch.

Insist that you massage your baby two or three times a day even when she is in the incubator. There are parents who have achieved results way beyond the expected development of a premature baby because of massage. By the way, don't be intimidated by all that medical apparatus. You can reach into the incubator and start massaging while talking to your baby in a way that assures her that you are there for her, and she will experience your presence and your love.

Despite the fact that premature babies have been subjects of many medical studies, few ever have the benefit of alternative therapies. Initiating touch very early is one sure way to help them on the road to a bright future.

If your baby was born with a brain injury and/or a birth defect, you are doubtlessly aware of all the life-saving techniques that modern medicine provides, yet the results of that trauma can last a lifetime. What better time to institute gentle massage to start counteracting the trauma?

Although their orientation to the premature population has grown in leaps and bounds in many areas, most physicians and nurses practice little in the realm of touch. Perhaps they are too busy. Perhaps they have yet to experience the amazing benefits of a loving touch.

HOW TO MASSAGE A PREMATURE BABY

Ask medical permission to put your hand in the incubator and gently stroke and or rub your baby. Give her little hands and feet a little squeeze. Place your hand on her diaphragm and feel her rhythm.

Help her experience the feeling of relaxing and breathing. One way to enhance breathing is to stretch her arms above her head, slowly letting go and then stretching again. This will start the chest muscles to function on their own.

You can also stretch her legs by putting one hand under the heel and the other on the thigh to stabilize the pelvis. Slowly stretch the leg, lengthening the hamstrings and forcing blood flow through the contracted muscles. Then bring the right knee up and stretch it over the left leg. Repeat on the other side. This will help loosen the legs from the pelvis and help the organs begin their vital functions.

Put your hand under the pelvis, and slide your hand down while you feel the pelvis relaxing. Then stroke your baby's chest and shoulders getting her to relax and breathe. When you are finished, give her little face and forehead a few loving strokes to emphasize how much you love her. Continue the touching and communicating until your baby leaves the hospital, no matter how long the stay is.

Remember that there is nothing stopping you from also introducing smells and different textures to your baby even at this tender age. The more stimulation, the more growth!

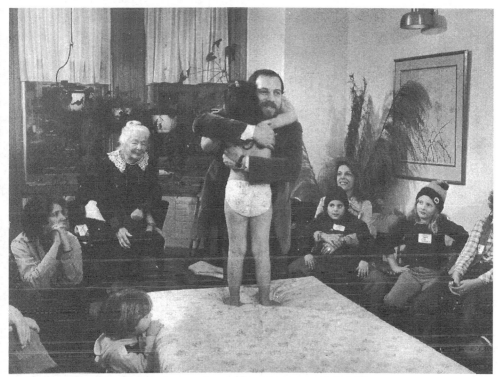
Dr Rolf and Robert Toporek beginning the Children's Project in Philadelphia.

In 1978, Dr. Rolf chose me to implement, manage, and complete a project to document, demonstrate, and promote the benefits of Rolfing for babies and children. There are many references throughout this book about Rolfing babies and children. Since 1975, I have Rolfed and documented over 300 families starting as early as day one and going as deep as four generations.

The Rolf Institute does not endorse my work with babies and children as of the publishing of this book but miracles never cease to amaze me. There are no books on Rolfing babies, children, and families. There is just what I learned by taking to heart Dr. Rolf's statement that she saw this as vital to the expansion of her life-long work and critical to the work itself. Rolfing babies and children, and my point of view, is not endorsed by anyone other than the people that have benefited from my work, but if you want to know more, feel free to contact me at teamchildren@teamchildren.com.

MY STORY

When I was little, my mother used to beat us with what was called cat-o'-nine tails. One day I provoked her so badly she took me out to the washroom in the back of our house and literally beat the hell out of me. I decided I would not let her know how much it hurt me, both physically and emotionally, and I held it in for years.

Later, during a tour of duty in Vietnam when I was eighteen years old, half of my squad was either wounded or killed, sometimes right in front of me. One day, one of my best friends, Milton Olive, who was the first African American to be awarded the medal of honor in the Vietnam War, was killed by a hand grenade thrown into a group of my squad members. I helped put his body back together, then wrapped it in a poncho and carried him out of the jungle. That first year, many of my friends were either killed or wounded. The mantra was "No, you cannot call your mother and go home. Suck it up and move on." When I returned home to a nation hostile to veterans, I chose to keep quiet about my experiences. In addition to the emotional trauma I experienced during these events, I also sustained physical damage with my rough-and-tumble approach. Little did I know that I would eventually find healing from both types of trauma through the therapeutic benefits of massage.

All things are connected in this life. In 1968, I returned home to Charleston, South Carolina, after having served two tours of duty in Vietnam. One of my first jobs was in a poverty program teaching low-literacy adults how to read, do math, and ultimately, get a job. Glamour magazine got word of my work and mentioned my name in an article.

My high school civics teacher, Miss Liddy (I would later drop out of high school and join the army), read the article, which ultimately led me to a woman Larkin Thompson.

Larkin told me about a fellowship from the Ford Foundation. I applied and in 1971 was given an unrestricted leadership development fellowship to study the methods and techniques of personal growth. During this time I met Will Schultz at a seminar in Georgia. He was based out of the Esalen Institute in Big Sur, California, where I showed up one day and announced my intention to become a group leader.

Again, one thing led to another, and it was at Esalen that Deborah Medows gave me my first massage. At one point in the massage, she shook my arm and told me to let go. I told her I had, but with a few gentle shakes, she told me to really let go. That was the first time I had ever experienced truly letting go, and I was profoundly moved by the power of touch. I owe a heartfelt thanks to Deborah and the many fine people I was privileged to meet and work with at Esalen.

Chief amongst these was Ida P. Rolf, founder of Structural Integration. I can honestly say that she was instrumental in helping me find my path in life. I was awestruck by her aura. My friend Sandy encouraged me to get a "Rolfing" session, and I ended up having three. My first few sessions with Seymor Carter were profound. In that moment, I decided to become a Rolfer and to learn under Dr. Rolf herself. In 1975, I was given that rare opportunity. Over the next four years, I was Dr. Rolf's East Coast business manager. I also lived and apprenticed with her son, Dick, and his family for over three years. Having found confidence in my ability, Dick and Bridget asked me to Rolf their youngest son, Michael. To know that someone trusts you is a happy feeling.

In 1978, Dr. Rolf chose me to implement, manage, and complete a pilot project to demonstrate and document the benefits of Rolfing babies and children. The results were amazing, and I produced a monograph and award-winning documentary entitled The Promise of Rolfing Children. Since then I have continued to Rolf entire families, including children from as early as one day old (my son Bryan) all the way to age ninety-eight.

For a period of time my life was not going well. My wife and mother of my son, Bryan, decided she did not love me anymore and spent a year focused on getting into a neonatal intensive care unit to demonstrate the power of touch at this most critical stage. So one day I took my Rolfing table to one of the most impoverished neighborhoods in Philadelphia unannounced, set it up on the sidewalk among drug dealers and addicts, and asked, "Who wants a massage?" The project continues to this day. At the time, the neighborhood was filthy, so we began cleaning it up, built a playground, and distributed books and school supplies.

Most important was the effect this project had on my son, Bryan. When he was about six or seven, I brought him with me for the first time. That day he discovered what a hypodermic needle was and began to appreciate where we lived and what we had.

Just after he turned ten, his mother passed away from cancer. The night she passed away we were lying in bed and he said, "I just want to talk to her one more time." I hugged my son and gave him permission to grieve. A few months later as I was driving him to school, I decided that the only way I could survive having a ten-year-old without a mother was to reach outside our own struggles and focus on a bigger problem. My practice was at its lowest, and my finances, quite frankly, had tanked.

So I came up with the idea to distribute two thousand low-cost, refurbished computers to those in need by the year 2000. Ed Brooks, a man whose name I found in the yellow pages, was my fortieth call to Realtors. Thirty-nine had said no, but Ed said yes and donated a warehouse where we repaired and distributed the computers.

We ran the administrative side out of my apartment. One part of the project asked recipients to write letters explaining why they needed a computer and how having one would help them. Over the years, Bryan has helped me read the letters, and he continues to help with the project to this day.

Through those letters, all involved have realized the deep connectedness that runs throughout humanity, especially in difficult situations such as those involving loss.

Here is a letter we recently received:

To whom it may concern:

I live with my husband and 1½- and 2½-year-old children. I lost my full-time job in February. My husband had been staying home with the children to save money on day care, so I was our only source of income. I am currently receiving unemployment, but it's only $201 a week, and our rent is $700 a month. We've mailed in an application for SNAP benefits, but we haven't received anything in regard to an interview or approval.

We're not currently receiving any assistance other than WIC, and we've had to go to food pantries to feed ourselves and the kids. We visited BirthRight, but they were only able to give us twelve diapers per child for the month, and we used those in less than a week. We've been using clothing diapers as much as possible; however, laundry detergent is just as expensive as diapers. We haven't been able to buy wipes since March. We're just using washrags every time we change the kids. After we pay rent, we literally have $104 left. I've maxed out all my credit cards and can't get approved for any more, nor can I get a loan. I'm having a tough time finding a new job because my previous employer made me sign a noncompete form upon being hired, so I'm not able to work in the same industry for a year (until next February).

We've rolled coins, drained our savings, returned cans and bottles, sold every piece of personal property we could get anyone to buy (including my cell phone). I feel so ashamed asking for help. Before I lost my job, I was making $2,000 a month salary and then between $4,000–$6,000 in commission depending on how busy the store was. My family live comfortably, bills were always paid on time and I never worried about how I was going to feed my kids let alone if I could afford their diapers.

I've never been in this position, and I've applied to every job not in my previous line of work that I've seen. I send my résumé to at least fifty employers a day. I can't even get a job with a cleaning company. I'm a hard worker. I used to work sixty hours, and it was nothing for me. I've always been the first person to volunteer or donate to a charity. Last Christmas I adopted a number of families to buy presents for, each with four kids. I'm great at money management. I've managed to keep afloat until now, and I'm at the end of my rope. I don't know what else to do now. I need help.

Not for myself, because I'd go months without eating and just deal with it. But seeing my kids suffer and being unable to provide for them is breaking my heart. They're such sweet babies who don't deserve this, and I feel like I've let them down. I just finished filling out my FAFSA so I can go back to school and finish my degree in nursing. Having a computer, whether it's a laptop or desktop, is an essential for college students now, and unfortunately there is no way possible we can afford one right now. Currently I'm borrowing family members' and neighbors' computers daily just to send out my résumé and check my email. It's going to be nearly impossible to attend school and excel if I don't have a computer at my disposal. If you have any programs that offer free computers or low monthly payments, please let me know. Thank you so much in advance.

Just before my son's mother passed away, she started a program to help kids whose mothers had died. Today it's a nationwide program that continues to help kids when either of their parents passes away. (See http://www.familyliveson.org/)

And the best gift I've ever received was from Bryan's wife, Alex, who told me that my son was the most kind and generous person she had ever met.

These are just a few examples of how making a difference can transform your life and the lives of those around you. To find out more, please visit www.teamchildren.org and www.handsonparenting.org.

One day my client and friend Buz Teacher, a publisher at Running Press, started following my work with massage and Rolfing children living in one of Philadelphia's most drug-ridden and impoverished neighborhoods. He was impressed with the transformational possibilities of my work and the Rolfing techniques, and he asked me if I would write a book on massage for babies and children. My answer was yes. A few years later, the first version The New Book of Baby & Child Massage was published and quickly became a valuable resource for parents worldwide. Running Press eventually merged with other companies, but because the message is so important, Running Press turned rights over to me so that I could republish, rebrand, and take the book and concept in exciting, new directions and to an expanded audience.

My next big breakthrough came when I met Steve Harrison, from Bradley Communications in Broomall, Pennsylvania, and joined his Quantum Leap program. Through Steve's encouragement, the coaches at Quantum Leap, and new contacts, not only is this book being republished and rebranded, we are also launching new and exciting programs to expand our mission to make a difference for every baby, child, and their family. The proceeds from this book will help fund our mission.

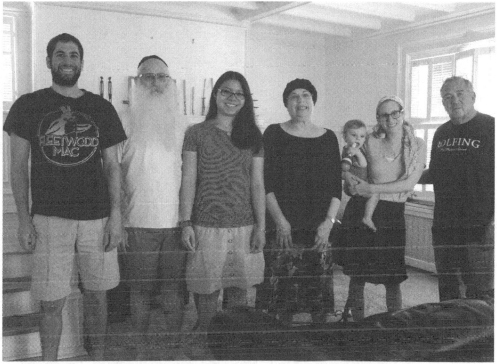

The Shinefields: Rolfing for three generations.

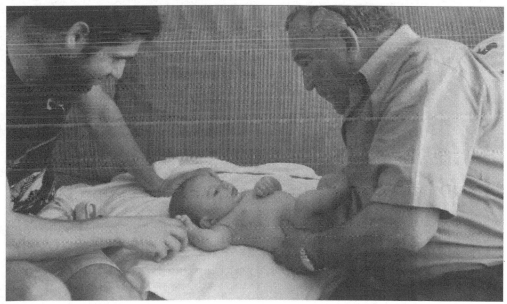

David and Akiva rolfing newborns.

TEAMCHILDREN.ORG

TeamChildren has evolved over time. Formerly known as "The Children's Project Inc.," it officially began in 1978 in Philadelphia. At the time, Ida Rolf wanted a way to demonstrate and document the benefits of her work with babies and children. I, on the other hand, wanted her to teach me how to work with babies and children. Initially, Dr. Rolf, a few other Rolfers, and I gathered in Philadelphia for a month, rolled up our sleeves, and went to work. Ron Thompson, a practitioner, took the photographs; Catharine Ellison provided some of the funding; and Carol Gold conducted interviews. The rest of us went to work with the babies and children who participated. Many others contributed in many ways. The results were remarkable.

Unfortunately, Dr. Rolf developed colon cancer and was unable to finish the project, so I took on the task of producing a monograph entitled "The Promise of Rolfing Children," which was published in 1981. A few years later I made the documentary The Promise of Rolfing Children, which focuses primarily on children with special concerns.

Since 1978, starting with Dr. Rolf's grandson Michael, I have Rolfed hundreds of babies and children as well as their entire families. About a dozen of these babies were only a few days old. The distinctions in this book came from what I learned during that time. It was also clear that for this project to make a real difference in the world, we would have to demonstrate the benefits of Rolfing, massage, and early stimulation on all children rather than just specific children.

In 1993, I began a project in one of the worst drug neighborhoods in the region, "The Badlands of North Philadelphia." I organized some volunteers, and we visited the area weekly. We set up tables on the sidewalk and offered massages to all the children. The results were truly amazing. However, through this experience we realized that the children in this neighborhood needed more than massage—they were starving for opportunities in all areas. We began by collecting and distributing books to the children, and finally computers.

Seeing the success of our computer program, I decided to expand it to the entire region. With the aid of volunteers, companies, individual donations, and a small staff, we have now helped distribute with minimal funding over fifteen thousand low-cost, refurbished computers to over seventy-five thousand kids in our region and beyond.

And we have loaded every computer with extraordinary software donated by www.brillkids.com, a company based in Hong Kong. We have also created a twenty-first-century early learning program in one of the largest preschool programs in Philadelphia.

With the republishing of Hands-on Parenting, a critical part of our effort, we will also be doing workshops and programs throughout the world.

TeamChildren is not a traditional organization and cannot be measured by what we have done or are doing. Dr. Rolf always emphasized that the whole is greater than the sum of its parts. Our mission is to plant and nourish the seeds of a human transformation, one in which we honor, respect, appreciate, and cherish the value and potential of each newborn and child. We want to help bring about a transformation where we as parents, communities, states, and nations give each child and family the tools, opportunities, and resources they need to succeed in life.

It is my intention that this book stimulate worldwide interest and funding in massage and in early neurological, cognitive, and social development. We are wholly committed to encouraging its universal acceptance and practice in a very short period of time.

If massage is so great, why isn't it universally practiced? Why don't doctors, hospital personnel, insurance companies, midwives, and nurses promote it? The answer is simple. Far too many people have never even had a massage and do not routinely get massaged, so they have no firsthand experience with how effective it can be for themselves and their children in general. They probably view massage as a luxury, not a necessity.

Remember, most everything we know about raising babies and children is based on the past and on maintaining tradition. This book, no doubt, has given you a whole new reality and body of knowledge in regard to raising your children. But why stop there? We want to improve, and to do so we'd like your input. Please stay in touch by writing or calling in care of TeamChildren.org, and let us know how this book has helped and how we can better present this material.

Like all great stories, we have no intention of this being the end, for you must realize by now that life is a continuum. This unfolding will help you and your children and possibly your neighborhood and community deal with and respond to the stresses of life in a healthier way. Just be sure to incorporate massage in your life and pass on the benefits to your family.

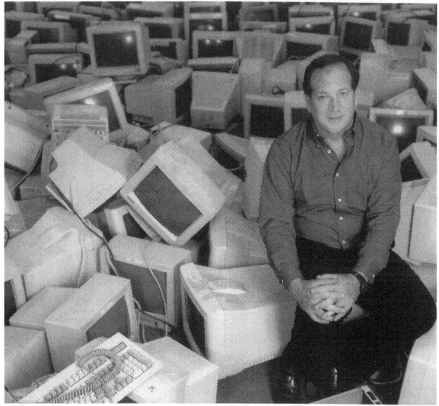

We have distributed over 15,000 low-cost high-quality refurbished computers loaded with amazing learning software reaching over 75,000 kids with minimal funding and staff. To contribute, visit www.teamchildren.org.

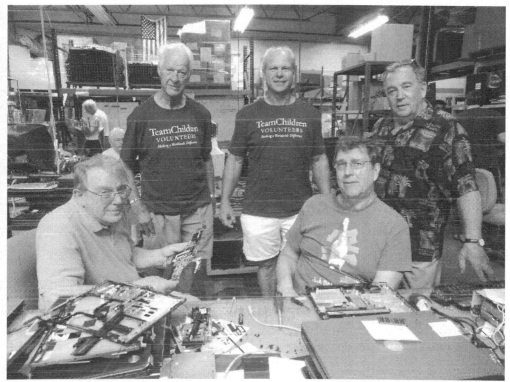

Team Children endorsed by Mark and Gordie Howe.

MOVING FORWARD

The money generated by the sale of this book will help fund our effort to bring this knowledge and its benefits to economically challenged children around the world. **To contribute, visit either www.teamchildren. org or www.handsonparenting.org**

The need for this book and its contents is critical for thousands and thousands of children around the world. In addition to making babies and children happier and physically healthier, it is just as important to massage their minds. From the moment of conception to age five, the brain is growing at a faster rate than at any other time in life. Because brain cells form in relation to the stimuli they are presented with, massaging a child's brain is as important as massaging their body. Smarter kids usually make better decisions. The world exists in language, and the more language you give a child, the more world they have.

As Benjamin Lee Worf puts it, "Language shapes the way we think and determines what we can think about."

In Chestnut Hill, Pennsylvania, the Institutes for the Achievement of Human Potential, founded by Glenn Doman, specializes in courses on early brain development. The institutes sponsor a one-week workshop called "How to Give Your Baby Encyclopedic Knowledge" and a one-week course on "What to Do about Your Brain-Injured Child."

I have taken these courses a number of times, and in addition to massaging and Rolfing my son, Bryan, from day one, we began using the tips and techniques highlighted after every section. By the time Bryan was one, he could read a thousand words and count to one hundred in English and Spanish. He could identify bits of information like "president," "primates," "polygons," and much more. By the time he was two and a half, he could turn a computer on and play learning programs like Reader Rabbit, Math Rabbit, Language Express, and many more. He read fluently by the age of three.

While there may be some who disagree with doing this with babies and children, I invite them to study the children I have worked with who have academically accomplished as much as Bryan or more. By the time Bryan was seventeen, he had graduated second in his high school class

124

and was one of the first four hundred kids accepted to Georgetown that year. After graduating from Georgetown, he worked for a number of years at www.edweek.org as an online news editor in charge of their social media, and he managed a blog on sports in education. By the time he was twenty-three, he had written so many blog posts on concussions in sports that they are now available as an eBook. On the side, he also wrote for Bleacher report and is now a senior copy editor.

A few years ago in China, I was introduced to KL Wong and the www.brillkids.com program. Because of my work with economically challenged families, KL has given us permission to install his early learning programs on the computers we distribute and to sell it at a reduced price on our www.handsonparenting.org website.

Many of the people reading this book may not be able to afford going to the institutes, take their courses or buy their products. For them we offer the Little Reader, Little Math, and Little Musician programs, all available for download on our website. These programs will make a huge difference.

A number of years ago we introduced this early brain development program in one of the largest preschool programs in Philadelphia. Unfortunately, we ran out of funding and could not continue. However, preliminary anecdotal comments from the parents showed that they loved what we had done with their children. We have followed up with a few of the kids, and they are now some of the top students in their classes. Google Aspira/TeamChildren on Youtube for some amazing videos.

Philadelphia has one of the biggest concentrations of poverty in the country. As of the publishing of this book, approximately 75 percent of the kids in the third grade in that city cannot read, write, or do math proficiently. This is true in many other schools throughout the country. We know the solution to this problem begins at home, and with the knowledge this book provides, it can end there. In a town not more than ten miles from my office, the infant mortality rate is double the surrounding counties. It is estimated that one out of four African American babies born there will die before the age of one. One of my goals is to demonstrate, then document how the knowledge in this book can help change that.

Please enjoy this book and the opportunity it will give you to take your parenting skills to new heights and the difference you can help us make for babies and children worldwide.

ORGANIZATIONS AND RESOURCES

www.handsonparenting.org

www.rolfingkids.org

www.teamchildren.org

www.rolfingtoporek.com

www.rolf.org

www.brillkids.com

www.brillbaby.com

www.iahp.org

www.landmarkworlwide.com

www.familyliveson.org

www.birthcenters.org

www.theiasi.net

www.rolfguild.org

www.hellerwork.com

www.anatomytrains.com

www.massage.com

www.amtamassage.org

www.massagemag.com

www.abmp.com/massage-and-bodywork-magazine

www.aap.org

ESALEN MASSAGE & BODYWORK ASSOCIATION HIGHWAY 1

www.esalen.org

TOUCH RESEARCH INSTITUTE

www.miami.edu/touch-research

INTERNATIONAL ASSOCIATION OF INFANT MASSAGE

www.iaim.net

OILS AND SUPPLIES

MASSAGE WAREHOUSE
www.massagewarehouse.com

BIOTONE
https://biotone.com/massage-products

BODYTHERAPY
wwwgotyourback.com

MASSAGE TABLES

OAKWORKS
www.massagetables.com

BLUE RIDGE TABLES
www.blueridgetables.com

CUSTOM CRAFTWORKS
www.customcraftworks.com

EARTHLITE
www.earthlite.com

STRONGLITE INC.
www.stronglite.com

PICES PRODUCTIONS
www.picespro.com

ULTRA-LIGHT CORP.
www.ultralightcorp.com

COMFORT CRAFT
www.comfortcraft.com

MAGAZINES

MASSAGE MAGAZINE
www.massagemag.com

ASSOCIATED BODYWORK & MASSAGE PROFESSIONALS
www.abmp.com/massage-and-bodywork-magazine

ABOUT THE AUTHOR

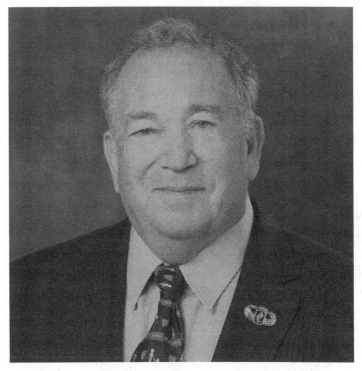

Robert Toporek is a Certified Advanced Rolf Practitioner who has helped over 4,500 men, women, and children transform their relationship to their bodies and lives. He is also the president and founder of TeamChildren, an international nonprofit organization with a mission to ensure that every parent has the tools, technology, training, and opportunity to help their children compete and contribute effectively in today's rapidly changing world.

Robert has been Rolfing since 1975 and continues to pioneer the benefits of Rolfing for babies, children, and families—which has been proven to improve posture, flexibility, and emotional connections, setting the groundwork for positive long-term results. He studied directly with Dr. Ida P. Rolf the last four years of her life and was her East Coast business manager. In 1978, Dr. Rolf chose Robert to implement and manage a project to demonstrate, document, and promote the benefits of Rolfing for babies and children.

Robert produced an award winning documentary and a monograph entitled *The Promise of Rolfing Babies and Children*. His goal is to substantially fund an effort to Rolf groups of babies and children and to document and promote those results worldwide. You can learn more at www.rolfingkids.org.

Through his work with TeamChildren, Robert has spearheaded an effort over the past 20 years to distribute refurbished computers to economically challenged children and their families, schools, and other nonprofit organizations. Without substantial funding or staff, they have distributed over 15,000 computers and reached over 75,000 kids.

Robert is a decorated Vietnam War veteran and served two tours of duty there from 1965 to 1967 with the 173rd Airborne Brigade Separate. During his first tour, he was awarded the Bronze Star with Valor, a Purple Heart, and the Vietnamese Cross of Gallantry with Palm Leaf. In his 2nd tour in Vietnam, he was the 2nd Battalion's non-commissioned officer in charge of the battalion's civil affairs program. In the refugee camp outside of his base camp, his team built a number of schools, a playground, a health center manned by volunteer doctors, , a boy scout lodge, and fed an orphanage weekly.

In addition to publishing and promoting this book, Hands-on Parenting, he is working on writing a book of Vietnam War stories. In the past few years he has begun to reunite with the people he served with in the weapons squad, third platoon of Company B, 2/503 Infantry, 173rd Airborne Brigade. Robert is the first Vietnam veteran to write a book on massage for babies and children. His transformation from warrior to healer is inspiring.

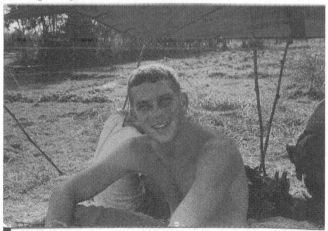

NOTES

1. Crystal Leonard, The Sense of Touch and How It Affects Development, http://serendip.brynmawr.edu/exchange/crystal-leonard/sense-touch-and-how-it-affects-development.

2. American Psychological Association, July 9, 2003, http://www.apa.org/research/action/massage.aspx.

3. Maria Konnikova, The Power of Touch, http://www.newyorker.com/science/maria-konnikova/power-touch.

4. Psychological Science, vol. 26, no. 2, February 2015, http://journals.sagepub.com/doi/abs/10.1177/0956797614559284.